THE ULTIMATE
SURPRISE

THE ULTIMATE SURPRISE

Jacqueline P. Jones

This book was printed in the United States of America.

To order additional copies of this book, contact:
Xlibris Corporation
1-888-795-4274
www.Xlibris.com
Orders@Xlibris.com
62539

CONTENTS

PROLOGUE

I am a "SURVIVOR". Even though everyday is still a challenge, I can truly say that I am a survivor. The purpose of writing "The Ultimate Surprise . . . Brain Tumor" is to express what affects this surprise and unexpected visitor had on my life and the lives of my family and friends. I am sure everybody probably thought that this was something really bad because there are very few of us who knew someone with a brain tumor. I, myself, always thought that if you had a brain tumor, that would be the end of your life. You can just imagine what thoughts were going through my mind.

It was very painful for me when I had to tell my family and friends about the tumor. After breaking the news to them, there was never a dry eye. I, myself, shed so many tears in those few days than I had in a long time. Trust me, I am a very emotional person to other's feelings and for this to make me this emotional took some getting used to because I was shedding these tears for myself. I've always had a shoulder for people to lean on and cry on and now it was my turn to do just that. I didn't really cry on everybody's shoulder but I had quite a few people to tell about this ultimate surprise.

You just cannot imagine how difficult it was for me to tell people that I had a brain tumor; yes a brain tumor! The first question most would ask is, "How did you find out about it?" I would answer that I didn't discover this myself. The results came from the doctor and an MRI. After answering this inquisitive question, most would say, "I'll be praying for you that everything will turn out okay'. I did tell everybody that it was a benign tumor because I knew that was on their minds but they just didn't know how to approach it because of the sensitivity of the tumor itself. They were relieved in that revelation. I told them that prayer was always welcome and I accept all prayers that would be said for me. How could I go wrong with the magnitude of prayer? I couldn't.

Okay, another purpose of this book is that I, Jacqueline Jones, asked God for a financial blessing because things were getting worse financially for my husband and me. After not being able to make ends meet (unaware of the recession), we were in dire straits. We prayed everyday and the Lord was listening and I knew I had to make a move.

So, one day Elroy and I were discussing the possibilities of reaching out to others by seeking groups to speak to about the tumor and the role it played in our lives. He was very adamant in his quest to spread the word about the tumor and how it affected our lives so drastically. As we were talking, it struck me as I was listening to him that I should write a book. The thought just bounced in my head from nowhere. This was not anything I was contemplating, especially after still suffering from the after affects of the surgery. I then asked him what his thoughts were about me writing a book. He looked at me in amazement and asked me if I really thought I could do that with all that I'd been through. I told him that he knew I could do anything that I set my heart and mind to and this was something that I felt I had to do for us. He then said, "Let's do it!" That was all the encouragement I needed. Henceforth, this is the beginning of the financial blessing that is going to be worthwhile for me writing this book. This tumor was not a planned event. It was an unforeseen surprise that ultimately affected our lives dramatically.

This is my purpose for "The Ultimate Surprise . . . Brain Tumor" and I hope that as you are reading this book, you will get a better understanding of a benign brain tumor (Meningioma) and the affects it will have on you and your family if you or a loved one is diagnosed with one.

This is a journey with many bumps in the road, and you may feel that as you progress and heal, the bumps are bumpier and the pain is unbearable, but as the journey will continue, the bumps will be easier to travel because the road will be so much smoother.

Before finding out about this ultimate surprise, I was serving as President of the Hampton Roads Chapter of Executive Women International®. The mission statement of this organization is:

Executive Women International® is an organization which brings together key individuals from diverse businesses for the purpose of:

- Promoting member firms

- Enhancing personal and professional development, and

- Encouraging community involvement.

The Hampton Roads Chapter was chartered in May 1987 and at the time of my role as President, there were 25 member firms. With today's economic situation, that number is less today due to the loss of several firms but we are still thriving and trying to gain new members. This organization helps a lot of women by being the leading connection to business professionals worldwide. My involvement with EWI® has enhanced my professional development tremendously and I am honored to be a part of such a prestigious group. The Norfolk Airport Authority® holds the membership in the organization and I am the representative.

The support I received from this organization was remarkable. It made going through this "ultimate surprise" easier to bear knowing that these ladies were there for me through all of the ups and downs, the trials and tribulations and the final recovery period.

With the diversity of women in this organization, I was able to connect with a dentist who has been giving me total dental care along with compassion and understanding about this ultimate surprise. There are so many wonderful people who have become a part of my life during this ordeal. Dr. Lynnette Young, who owns Young Family Dentistry is a very caring dentist. I am not a dentist lover and always have had a fear of that office visit, but through the radiation treatments and the numbness I still feel, I thought it was time to conquer that fear and face the dentist. Well, it really wasn't a bad experience because she has such a caring staff and everybody is treated like royalty (special) which makes it easier to bear whatever news that might come your way and more prepared to face the treatment plan established just for you. Now, that's special.

I knew I was going to face some challenges and was ready to conquer them teeth first. Well, those challenges are coming to an end when I have that beautiful smile that I've always wanted. Thanks to Dr. Young and her staff, my dream is coming true. You will get a chance to see my smile when we meet.

Words cannot express the gratitude I have for them as women and friends. They are considered life-long friends as far as I am concerned.

CHAPTER 1

The Ultimate Surprise— Meningioma (Brain Tumor)

This chapter will take you through the beginning of the ultimate surprise. This is a story worth sharing and I want to be the one to do it. This is a very painful experience and the pain just don't want to go away after surgery. I pray that it will eventually disappear but I'm not quite sure that it will. I will now take you on the journey of the ultimate surprise.

Have you ever experienced a headache on one side and just wished that it would please go away? This headache was on my right side mainly over the eye. On April 5, 2008, I had that experience. Now, I am not the type of person who would normally get headaches, especially an excruciating one that was a constant companion the entire weekend. I've had my share of sinus headaches but this was no comparison to a sinus headache. Coupled with the headache was the double vision I was experiencing in my right eye since the middle of March. I was sure in my mind that it was coming from not visiting my Ophthalmologist and I was overdue for my yearly eye exam. My daughter and husband urged me to seek emergency medical attention at one of our local Urgent Care Centers over the weekend, but I felt that I could wait to call my primary care physician on Monday, April 7, which I did. I felt that I had suffered enough over the weekend and could hardly wait for Monday to make that call.

I called my doctor's office on Monday and found out that he was not in that day so the receptionist scheduled my appointment for the next day, which was Tuesday, April 8, 2008. When I went in for my appointment, I told the doctor about my headaches. He did some examinations and asked me how long I had the headaches and the double vision. He really didn't't say a lot but ordered an MRI "stat". I guess that meant he wanted to see immediately what was going on inside my head. Well, he didn't have to wait too long. On Thursday, I received a call from his office that he needed to see me the next day which was Friday, April 11, to give me the results of my MRI. I was wondering what he had to tell me that he couldn't tell me over the phone. I've been seeing him for quite a few years and I knew something wasn't right if he would prefer to see me rather than calling me on the phone.

The reason I say this is because in June 2007, I was scheduled to have surgery (hysterectomy) and the day before the surgery, after I had cleansed my entire system out, I got a call from him to tell me that I could not have the surgery due to the creatnine level in my kidneys. He said that if I chose to still have the surgery, I would wake up on dialysis. Now, that was a real wake-up call and needless to say, the surgery was postponed until August 2007 when the levels were much improved. He took care of this bad news over the phone, so I was wondering what this could be that I had to make a trip back to his office.

The thought that was going through my mind was the fall that took place with me in 2002. While going down a flight of stairs, I tripped, fell down and hit the cement floor really hard. During the fall, I sustained some severe injuries (fractured left wrist and ankle and sutures over my left eye) and I was out of work for 6 weeks during the healing process. I thought that this was a result of that 5 years later. All sorts of thoughts go through your mind when you are facing the unknown and the thought of being called into the doctor's office for results from a test that he ordered didn't make you feel any better. I am always a positive thinking person and the thought of a brain tumor never entered my mind. To be truthful, no thoughts were entering my mind. I drew a blank and was just going to wait for the outcome from the doctor.

Needless to say, I went to see him on April 11 and he gave me some very alarming news. My daughter was there with me to ease her mind as well as my pain. He had the results in his hand and he read it to me. He read the report that stated:

Reason for Exam: Double Vision

History: Right sided headache and diplopia for one week. History of diabetes and hypertension.

Diagnostic Interpretation:

Findings: "MRI of the brain was performed using standard pre- and post-gadolinium protocol pulse sequences. There is no diffusion. A well circumscribed, extra-axial mass, measuring 2.4 cm X 2.2 cm, demonstrates prominent homogeneous enhancement, located subjacent to the inferomedial right temporal lobe with associated mass effect and the suggestion of a dural tail along its anterior aspect of axial images. This mass is essentially isointense to gray matter on unenhanced and long-TR image sequences. Hyperintense signal is seen on long-TR images in the adjacent right temporal lobe suggestive of associated edematous changes in this region. The optic chiasm and both nerves are normal in caliber with no abnormal signal intensity or evidence of atypical enhancement. The cerebrospinal fluid spaces are normal for age. The midline structures are unremarkable. Flow voids are present in the major vessels at the base of the brain. Evidence of a remote left orbital wall blowout fracture with herniation of left retro-bulbar fat medially and growing through no entrapment, of the adjacent left medial rectus muscle. Otherwise, the extracranial soft tissues are unremarkable".

Impression: "Enhancing 2.4 cm X 2.2 cm in the extra-axial right temporal lobe, most suggestive of a meningioma. Other extra-axial masses are feasible though thought to be less likely. No associated direct invasion or abnormal signal is currently seen in the adjacent optic nerve or optic chiasm".

After having read the report, he said you have a meningioma. I really did not know what that was. He finally said that it was a "tumor" and it must be removed. After I heard that word "tumor", I didn't hear anything else but was thinking "Oh my God!! A Tumor?!?" "A Brain Tumor?!?". That was definitely and truly my "ultimate surprise". It was an ultimate surprise because I had no idea that this could happen to me but I thank God that my daughter was there to help me absorb this news and surprise. She is really strong and can understand most of the doctor's statements and ask questions. While we were there, he immediately used his cell phone to call a surgeon. Can you imagine your doctor placing a call from his cell phone? Things have really changed with this modern technology. He stepped out of the examination room to talk but the surgeon was not available and couldn't be reached at the moment. He left a message for him to call him back. In the meantime, I had an appointment with the Ophthalmologist that same day and we had to leave to get to that appointment.

All sorts of thoughts were racing through my mind as my daughter and I were going to my other appointment. We were wondering why this was happening to me and what the outcome would be if I had to have surgery. I was a bundle of nerves and just could not think straight at the moment. I knew I had to see the Ophthalmologist who would probably have more bad news for me. I just could not concentrate on anything but that "tumor" that was in my head and giving me lots of trouble and pain. What a trying time this was and all I could do was to try not to cry but it was getting very difficult to hold back those tears. I didn't want to put more pressure on my daughter so I had to be strong for the both of us even though I was a bundle of nerves inside. It was like being in a well just before you hit the water and once you hit the bottom, you realize that the well is dry. I know this might sound strange, but if you were to get the news that you had a brain tumor, what kinds of thoughts would you have? It's really hard to imagine what you might think if you were faced with this same situation. Trust me, the thought of your mortality definitely comes to mind, but you can't let those thoughts consume your ability to think about the positive things in your life such as family and friends. My thoughts were on my grandchildren and how they would grow up to be adults. I knew I wanted to be a part of their lives a lot longer to see them change over the years. I love them very much and just could not bear the thought of not being around them. Those are the kind of thoughts I was having, along with the possibility of surgery. I just could not imagine how surgeons could open your head, remove a foreign article, close your head back up and send you home. That was an amazing thought that I was constantly thinking about.

My appointment with the Ophthalmologist was very unusual because there wasn't much he could do since my double vision had gotten worse. My primary care physician had already called him so he knew, as well as his staff, what was going on. It's really amazing how people treat you when they know certain things about you. It's as though they want to reach out to you but just don't know how to do it at the time. While they are trying to put your mind at ease, you can see the worry and stress on their faces as if they are saying "I feel sorry for you" without actually saying it. That's the way I saw it when I went in to see the doctor.

He ordered me to do some field tests as well as dilate my eyes for an examination. After the examination, he requested that I come back to him after the surgery so he could do another examination without the double vision. He took a picture on his instant Polaroid camera and put it in my file. He showed it to me but I really didn't know the significance of that picture except it showed my eyes that didn't look very healthy at the time. I did know that my head was still hurting really bad and I was ready to go home and lie down. He referred to the double visions as diplopia which was the term that was used in my MRI interpretation. So, I learned quite a few new words for the day which still didn't make me feel any better. I was still faced with the unknown of this ultimate surprise.

By the time I had returned home from my appointments, the surgeon's office, Dr. Joseph Koen, had called to let me know when my appointment was going to be with him. It was scheduled for Wednesday, April 17, 2008. In the meantime, I had to break this news to my husband. I did not want to wait until he was off from work so I took a chance and called him on his cell phone and he answered. I couldn't ease the blow when I told him and his first response was, "you're kidding". I immediately told him that this was not anything I would kid about because this was very serious.

He told me that he would see me when he got home. I then called my boss to tell him and he was shocked, too. I know that everybody that I told was shocked and it didn't make it any easier to tell them. The weekend of this ultimate surprise was spent feeling more pain and breaking the news to my family, especially my mother. She was devastated when I broke the news to her but I reassured her that I would be okay and I would keep her posted of any developments, especially after I visited the surgeon. I think she tried to feel better so I wouldn't worry.

The pain and the double vision were getting worse but I knew I had to get myself together to go to work on Monday and wait for the doctor's visit on Wednesday. To be at work after telling my bosses of this ultimate surprise was strange. I went in Mr. Scott's office and asked Mr. Shank to join us. It was an awakening experience to talk to them and let them know how I felt. I was very scared and uncertain about what the surgeon would tell me. I conveyed these feelings to them and they reassured me that they would stand by me throughout this ordeal and that made me feel better and to realize even more that this was one of the best places to work. I am, today, very fortunate to have them as bosses. In today's society, it is hard to find bosses that genuinely care for your well-being and are willing to work with you through your health issues, but they beat all odds.

Today is Wednesday and it is time to see Dr. Koen, the surgeon. At this appointment, my husband and daughter were both able to accompany me because we knew this was going to be a very important appointment. We also knew that we would get some much needed answers and explanations on this ultimate surprise tumor. When we met with the surgeon, after the introductions were made, he immediately showed us the film from the MRI which he had displayed out in the hallway adjacent to the examination room. We had to bring the film with us for this visit. We were able to see where this mass was in my head as well as the tail that was attached to it. It is really amazing to see your brain on film. It is also scary, too, to see a tumor that want to take over your brain. To think that this invasion is inside your head near your brain, the central nervous system in your body can send a healthier person over the edge. I was petrified. The surgeon also pointed out that my brain was beginning to swell, which we also saw on the film. That was really amazing to see your brain looking oversized in your head. It was clearly visible that it was swelling. It was looking like it had no space to breathe or think. He was very concerned about the swelling and knew that something had to be done expeditiously or it was going to keep swelling. My thoughts were if it kept swelling, would there be a possibility of it bursting? In my state of mind, every weird thought that I could think of came to me. I was devastated to actually see this tumor with its tail in my head. To tell the truth, I almost lost it and, once again, my daughter and husband had to speak for me as well as absorb all the surgeon was saying. I could see the worried looks on their faces as well as on mine, but they had to be strong for me because I was just too weak to do anything myself. I did ask him when can he remove it. I knew within myself that I wanted this invasion in my head removed because it had no place in my life or in my head. I felt like it was the enemy and I had to defeat it before it invaded other parts of my body. That is the way I was thinking yet telling myself that I had to still be rational.

He informed us that he would try to remove all of the tumor but was concerned with the tail attached to it. We could clearly see it on the film as he pointed it out to us. He did not want to invade a territory that was too dangerous and would have life changing consequences, but he would do his best. He said he would have to order another MRI after the surgery to see exactly what he couldn't remove and determine the best way to combat the remains. He said it would probably be radiation treatments. This was way too much information to absorb at the present time, but we were grateful that he explained everything in such in-depth detail. He informed us that he had just gotten a cancellation from one of his patients that was having surgery the following Friday, April 25, 2008 and if I was interested in that date, it was okay with him. I told him that if it was alright with him, I would take that spot. He also informed me that I would have to be at the hospital at 5:30 a.m. the morning of the surgery because I would be the first one that day. Needless to say, we did not hesitate to tell him that we would be there. His office then set up my pre-operative appointments at the hospital (chest x-ray, EKG and several tubes of blood) which, I must tell you, are always required before you have surgery. They have to make sure that you are physically fit to undergo the surgery and how you will handle the anesthesia because we all know that you are between life and death while you are under the anesthesia.

I continued to work leading up to the day of my surgery. My bosses did not particularly want me at work because they felt that the tumor might burst. It was a very trying time for them and I think they really didn't know how to approach me to tell me to stay home until the surgery. I really wasn't feeling good the week leading up to my surgery due to the pain I was experiencing and the double vision that was getting worse day by day. It was hard to focus at my computer because everything was doubled. It was also hard to write because the vision would make everything double which made it difficult to even sign my name. Nothing would focus clearly. I decided that it would be best that I stop working two days before the surgery to put everyone's minds at ease, including mine. I was having more affects from the tumor and it was getting scary. I felt that it was trying to take over my life and my well-being. I convinced myself that my main objective was to get it removed so I can go on with my life without it. I knew I was not going to miss it being a part of my life. As a matter of fact, I was ready to send it on its way to wherever it would go after its removal.

In the meantime, Dr. Koen ordered another MRI the Wednesday before my surgery on Friday. This was supposed to be the module he would use during the operation. It was supposed to be a 3-D module. Can you just imagine your face on a 3-D module? I would have loved to have seen that but, of course, that was not possible. My husband, daughter from Washington and my two grandsons went with me for this procedure. It was a lengthy process and I was feeling really bad and dizzy before, during and after the procedure. It was so bad that they had to roll me out of the imaging area in a wheelchair because my balance was not good and they did not want me to fall and injure myself. We had to wait for the technician to copy the CD which had to be taken to Dr. Koen's office after the imaging was done. We completed that task and headed home so I could get some much needed rest. My energy level these days was not good and rest was needed constantly.

I was now two days from surgery and I was getting anxious and scared at the same time. This is a surgery that I didn't know of anyone who had ever had it, so I was really facing the unknown from this ultimate surprise. I knew I couldn't ponder on the unknown but face it with full force and a positive attitude. I had prayers coming from across the United States so I was not worried about the outcome because I had the power of prayer and the Grace of God on my side. I was going in with true optimism that everything was going to be okay and I was going to be much better. Not as good as new, but okay. With those positive thoughts, how could I lose? There was no way I was going to lose this battle. My surgeon gave me assurances that everything was going to be alright and I trusted everything he said because he was the surgeon and these surgeries are performed by him regularly. He was the expert and I was the patient. He was going to have my life in his hands and I was convincing myself that there was not much to worry about once I went into the operating room. The power of prayer was also on my side. Again, how can I lose?

I mentioned my daughter and my two grandsons from Washington State accompanied me for the MRI. Well, when she heard the news about my tumor, she was very distraught and told her husband that she had to come and be with me. You see, she is the youngest of my two daughters and she and I are very close. Well, I am very close with both of my daughters. My oldest daughter is more like my rock. She keeps me focused and my youngest daughter is just that, my youngest daughter. Even though she is a wife and mother, she is still my youngest daughter. Her husband is in the Navy and they have programs to help families who need to travel home for illnesses and other emergency reasons. The Navy was able to get her and the kids a plane ticket to come to Virginia to be with me during my surgery. They arrived April 19, 2008, which was the Saturday before the surgery date of April 25. I had just been out to Washington in February to await the birth of my grandson on February 8, 2008. I was the chosen one to be in the delivery room with her and to even cut the cord. That was an exciting event which I will never forget. That was an awakening experience that I wouldn't have dreamed could happen to me (just like the ultimate surprise?). I was very thankful to have had that opportunity to be with my daughter during this time. I will never forget that experience and I have pictures to remind me of it. I was doubly pleased when I was able to meet her and the kids at the airport where I work. Jameka and Adrianna were there, as well, and we were all waiting together for their arrival. That was an occasion I did not want to miss so I made that sacrifice to be there when they came down the concourse. The smiles on their faces were more than Kodak moments. I was amazed at how much my youngest grandson, Joshua, had grown and he was only two months old. It's also amazing how much babies change from month to month. He was a very happy camper because he smiled at everybody. Those smiles made me feel very good inside. Xavier, my oldest grandson, who is my buddy, was very happy to see us. He brought us up to speed about what he had been doing since we last saw him. We were all very happy to be together again even under these circumstances. Family is very important to me and to have my immediate family in my presence was more than phenomenon. It was awesome. We could spend some family time together and catch up on everything that had been going on in our lives. It's amazing how little tid-bits of information can mean so much to you at certain times in your life.

Chapter 2

Day of Surgery

Okay, let's get back to this brain tumor and the ultimate surprise. The thought of someone opening your head, cutting through your skull to get to the Menangioma is enough right there for an ultimate surprise. I will take you through the process from start to finish as I was told and as I remember for this day of surgery:

★ Arrive at hospital at 5:30 a.m. to check in. I had to make my co-pay at the time of admission.

★ After admission and signing all the paperwork, I was immediately taken in the back for vital signs and was advised that the MRI I had taken 2 days before was not sufficient for the surgeon and was not what he ordered, so he had scheduled another one for 6:00 a.m. the morning of surgery. We were at awe because I had to pay a $100 co-pay for that MRI and he couldn't use it after I waited for the CD to take to him afterwards. This was very upsetting and disappointing, too. There wasn't anything we could do because it was the day of surgery and we did not want to delay that any further. I also knew that I could not get upset to raise my blood pressure which would delay the surgery further. Things happen for a reason and who was I to question an MRI when I am just the patient awaiting surgery. I kept my mind opened and my feelings in tact. I would worry about this later after the surgery

★ After getting undressed and putting on the hospital gown, I was prepped for the IV that was started as well as getting my blood sugar checked since I am a diabetic, also. I was informed that someone would be taking me down for the MRI very soon. My husband was with me when this was told to me so he went to tell my waiting family members and dear friend, Debbie Meads, the news and this would most likely delay my surgery because this will take about 30 minutes.

★ I was wheeled down for the MRI which took approximately 30 minutes and then I had to wait additional time for someone to come get me and take me back downstairs.

★ Once I came back to the surgery waiting area, the anesthesiologists came in to go over my medical record and to ask me several questions about my diabetes and the bronchitis I had in February (2 months ago) that pertained to my health. I explained the bronchitis which was a result from my trip to Washington State but everything was better and I didn't have any effects from it at this time. This put their mind at ease as well as the blood sugar test they performed which was good. I was glad that I didn't have to push my panic button. I had just overcame another obstacle along my way to surgery. During this time, Dr. Koen made his entrance also, to make sure everything was still a "go" and after everyone had went over all of the vitals and my history, we were finally ready to proceed to the operating room.

★ I remember the ride to the operating room and that is all I remembered until I woke up in the ICU.

Waking up in the ICU was an experience in itself. I remember the oxygen being administered to me through an oxygen mask. The air was very cool. As I can recall, I had some pain when I woke up, which was not as bad as I thought it would be. My head was bandaged and I was very groggy and sleepy. I also remember members of my family speaking to me and just to hear their voices and see their smiles, I knew I had made it through one of the most serious operations imaginable. I recall thinking to myself that this was a new day for me, almost like a rebirth because this day was the beginning of a new outlook on life. I can remember thinking that while coming from under the anesthesia and being able to open my eyes was truly a blessing. My family and friends were allowed to come in to see me in intervals and for very short periods of time. I managed to see everyone that was there, especially my family that traveled from North Carolina to be with me before, during and after the surgery. There was a total of 14 waiting for my outcome in the waiting room and that went a long way with me and the surgeon. He was amazed that so many people were there to support me. I was amazed, too, that my family would travel from North Carolina to be there during my surgery. Everybody knew the seriousness of this type of surgery and they wanted to be there to see the outcome. Needless to say, they were pleased. My sister, her daughter and grand daughter came the night before the surgery. They provided me inspiration and spiritual blessings to carry into the operating room. They were there at the hospital at 5:30 a.m. on the day of surgery. My dear friend, Debbie Meads (who will tell anyone that she is my twin), was also there at 5:30 a.m. that morning. Her main objective was to be with my husband and to cater to his needs because he was a nervous wreck. Everyone also tried to keep him as calm as possible. I heard he did a lot of pacing and walking during this time, but he never said a word. They knew what he was going through and just let him be in his own world when he needed to be there. I also heard that my grandchildren were on their best behavior through the ordeal of waiting. I know they were probably wondering where Grammy was, but they were content and played with each other during the wait time. I was very proud of them and pleased that they did so well under the circumstances.

Once Dr. Koen came out with the news, everyone was happy that I had come through without any complications. I am sure I was happy, too, but didn't know it yet. This was major surgery and I made it through to tell about it. The surgery took longer than anticipated due to the location of the tumor and the difficult in trying to extricate it. The surgeon told the family that he tried to get it all but don't think that he did. He would order another MRI to see what is left. If there is any of the tumor (the tail) left, he would order radiation treatments to eventually kill the remaining cells.

I think the craniotomy took the longest time because of the reconstruction after the surgery. Craniotomy is a cut that opens the cranium. During this surgical procedure, a section of the skull, called a bone flap, is removed to access the brain underneath. The bone flap is usually replaced after the procedure with tiny plates and screws. In my case, the surgeon informed me that some of the bone had broken and therefore, they had to use some type of cement along with the titanium screws to get it back together. Now that was amazing to hear that I might have cement in my head also. Also, have you ever heard the term: "do you have any screws loose?" Now, I can honestly say, "I'll have to check that out". I guess I can really make light of this situation with some humor. I wonder if anyone was going to ask me if my head felt heavy due to the cement. Who knows what sort of questions, comments and jokes I will encounter but I will be ready with my come-back.

I am convinced that I made it through this major surgery because I had a number of people throughout the United States praying for me. It was God's hands that guided my surgeon and his team while I was in that operating rom. I know this and I believe this. I am a living testimony of what God can do for you if you believe in His power and have faith. I don't mind sharing my experience with anybody who will listen to me.

I can still remember that, being in ICU, you are given extra attention because they need to know how you are doing after this major surgery. The nurses would come in about every 20 minutes to check my vital signs and to get my pain ratio which ranged from 1-10, with 10 being the highest threshold for pain. If I said my pain was at 10, they would immediately administer more pain medication through my IV. They also asked me the same questions every time they came to check on me. The questions were:

★ Do you know where you are?

★ What year is it?

★ What is your name?

★ Can you squeeze my hand?

I had no problem complying with their questions. I knew these were tests that were required after brain surgery and I also knew

I had to pass these tests in order to be discharged to go home. I was also told afterwards that I was doing a great job and the nurses always smiled. I knew I had to be the best patient possible and that is what I was doing.

During the first night in ICU, I think I slept okay. I remember my throat being extremely sore due to the breathing tube that was placed in before surgery and was removed after surgery while I was still under the anesthesia. It was a pleasure to know that I didn't wake up with it still inserted because I was told by the surgical staff that it could be a possibility that the tube would still be in if there were any complications during surgery. The nurse gave me something to drink and it was very hard to swallow but I did it. I was having bouts of nausea and I let the nurse know that. She gave me something to make it go away and I rested the remainder of the night.

I was awakened during the night for the nurse to check me for MRSA which is a type of Staph bacteria that can cause very serious bacterial infections. MRSA stands for Methicillin Resistant Staphylococcus Aureus and there are no vaccinations for this bacterial infection. There had been some cases reported at this hospital so this was a precaution they do on each patient. The procedure was simple and painless because she swabbed the inside of my nose with a long Q-tip and that was it. I was informed later that the test was negative so I was happy about that because a Staph infection would not have been good for me or anybody for that matter. Any type of infection after surgery is not good and that is why they give you antibiotics in your IV to fight those germs that might want to invade your body. Luckily, I was germ-free during my stay at the hospital. That meant I would not have to stay an extended period of time to fight off any infections. That made me feel really good to know I would be closer to going home sooner.

I know I was not a pretty sight after the surgery due to the turban bandage I had on my head and the swelling as well as the right eye being closed. I couldn't see the bandage, but I knew it was there because I could feel it on my head. It felt sort of heavy and bulky but with what I was going through, that was the least of my concerns. My husband said I was the most beautiful sight to him because he was thankful that I came through the surgery. As far as he was concerned, just seeing me was all that mattered. He thanked the Lord for bringing me through the surgery and back to him.

I was hearing these noises in the back of my head that sounded like waves of water. With my vision in the right eye; it was still doubled but the colors I was seeing were green and purple. I don't know why those were the colors but I guess it had something to do with the optic nerves and the possibility of damage caused by the tumor. I mentioned this to the surgeon and he said it was coming from the tumor and it should soon go away. I trusted his answer and just hoped for the best. I didn't dislike those colors so I just dealt with it. It was just strange to look at someone and they were purple and green.

CHAPTER 3

The Day After Surgery

The next morning, I had breakfast. It was painful to open my mouth to eat but I had to eat to regain my strength. The nurse assisted me with my breakfast and helped me to get through this painful ordeal. Once I ate a little, I felt like I had renewed strength and was ready to see Dr. Koen. He made his round and told me how good I looked after having surgery. He told me that I did good throughout the operation but he was unable to remove all of the tumor (the tail). He reminded me of the MRI that he showed us at my first visit in his office and the tail that was attached to the tumor. Well, that still remains and he will talk to me later about what options to take. I wasn't able to quite comprehend what he was saying so I let my husband and daughter carry on with him while I was still trying to recuperate enough to go home. That made me feel good because even though he said I looked good, I didn't really feel good because I was swollen and with my right eye, which didn't want to stay open for long periods of time, I was still seeing the different colors when my eye was open. The colors I was seeing were still green and purple. Now, I don't know why those were the colors of choice for my right eye, but that was what I was seeing. Also, there was a sound I was hearing coming from the back of my head. It was like pulsating water flowing and I just could not shake it. I guess that was part of the craniotomy that was performed. At the time, I did not know this, but found out about this later on. To think that your scalp was cut open to expose your skull and then your skull was sawed open to cut through the protective lining to reach your brain is amazing. I could not imagine lying on a table with my head anchored to a table while this procedure was being performed, but I finally came to the realization that this really happened and I can live to tell about it. Even though there was quite a lot of pain,

I can live to tell about it. Even though the pain was so severe that I couldn't think straight, I can live to tell about it. What an ultimate surprise to tell.

This is still the day after surgery (Saturday) and I was still in ICU. There was a schedule for visitors while you are in ICU. There was only certain times for visitors and the visit time was about 15 minutes. I did have several visitors that day as I can recall. I was glad that some friends came to visit even though I was not looking my best, but it was good to know that friends will come to visit you while you are in the hospital and could care less what you look like. They were just happy that I came through the surgery and could still remember who they were. Most of my friends did not know what to expect when they walked into my room. I was not hooked up to a lot of machines and could hold a conversation with them and even laugh at some of their comments. They were really pleased of this outcome and could hardly wait to pass it along to other friends who could not come visit me in the hospital. I was happy to see them and enjoyed their visits.

As I got through the second day after surgery, the hospital provided hygiene services which was very unusual to have someone to come in to give you a bath. I mean literally give you a full scale bath. The lady was an older lady and was very gentle and caring. She asked my husband to leave the room while she performed her duty. It was good to have a bath after being in the hospital for two days and having had surgery. She really knew what she was doing and I soon got over my shyness and just let her do what she was good at doing. After she finished, I was squeaky clean and ready to go to sleep, which I did. I had more visitors that day and Elroy stayed until night fall when I insisted that he go home to get some rest. He was really tired and worn out, so he didn't put up much hesitation and left. When he left, I missed him, but knew that he needed his rest because it has been a very trying time for him and my daughter and grandsons were there to keep him company. I was wishing that I could go home with him but I knew I had to be patient and wait for Dr. Koen to discharge me.

During the middle of the night, the nurse came to inform me that I was being transferred from ICU to a private room. It was amazing to be removed at 1:30 a.m. to another ward. I was placed in a wheelchair and wheeled to my room. I met the new nurses and was very pleased with their kindness. I was helped to my bed and after all vitals were done, I was able to rest and get some more sleep. I was happy that I was recovering well enough to leave the ICU unit and was feeling really blessed at the time and thinking this was closer to going home soon. While you are in the hospital, you can only think about getting out of the hospital and going home. Those were the thoughts that stayed on my mind constantly while I was there.

CHAPTER 4

Day Three After Surgery

It was good to be in a private room at last. Even though I was in a private room in the ICU unit, this felt more like a real private room. The third day after surgery was Sunday and it was the day the bandage was to be removed. I had several visitors this day, too, and when the surgeon came in, he cleared the room so he could remove my "turban". I personally did not see it while it was on, but I saw it when he took it off and to my surprise, it was not very bloody. He was pleased with the closure of the incision with the 37 staples that it took. The incision was from the top of my forehead to the top of my ear. I could not quite comprehend or see what he was talking about because I did not have access to a mirror to see it. When my visitors came back in the room, they saw what I couldn't see and they just stared at my head. That made me feel uneasy and thought I might look like a monster or an alien. By me not being able to see what they saw, I just couldn't imagine what I looked like. I knew my eye was swollen shut and my face felt like it was swollen, too. I just didn't worry too much about it because I was glad I had friends and family with me to make me still feel good to be alive.

After going through this type of surgery, all kinds of thoughts go through your mind and you have lots of time to think about what exactly happened in that operating room while you were between life and death. That is time you can never get back or remember because once they put you under, everything else is oblivious to what is being done to you. You know you are in the best possible hands with all of the people that are in the operating room tending to your every need and keeping an eye on all of your vital signs. When you finally wake up, you are blessed to wake up and you just want to thank every team player for their caring ways to assist you with your breathing and to keep your body acclimated every second while the surgery is being performed; from the first incision to the last staple. It is good to know that these professional medical providers were there just for you. At this point and time, you are the most important person in the operating room and these team players were specially picked just for your care. Now, that really makes going through any type of surgery worthwhile. I must say that it is not something that I would look forward doing again.

Trust me, I was glad that surgery was an option for me to remove this tumor and I just couldn't imagine the idea of cutting my head open, sawing through my skull and exposing my brain. In my wildest dreams, this was not something I expected to happen to me, but it did. That, in my opinion, is the "ultimate surprise". I was very fortunate, that this type of tumor is benign and not cancerous. When you hear "brain tumor", the first thing that comes to mind is cancer. You always hear of people having brain cancer and I am very lucky and blessed that those words did not describe me. I can't sit back and keep asking "why did this happen to me?" or "I didn't ask for this to happen to me." I just can't feel sorry for myself because I have a long road ahead of me once I get out of this hospital and go home. I know the healing process is going to be long and I must stay strong to go through it, especially the pain.

The surgeon came by and informed me that if I keep doing like I'm doing, he will let me go home tomorrow (Monday). I was happy to hear that news because there is no place like home and even though I was getting excellent care in the hospital, I was ready to go home to be in my own surroundings. I know in the back of my mind that this wasn't going to be easy, going home three days after a major surgery like that. My family did not think that was a good idea, but the doctor knows best. They thought that the doctor didn't go through the surgery, so how could he make this decision three days after surgery. I did not argue with the doctor because I, myself, was ready to go home, so I agreed with his decision. I knew how I felt and I felt like it was time for me to go home and start my recuperation because, again, there is no place like home and I was ready for the challenges that I had to face.

CHAPTER 5

Going Home Day

This is the day I go home, Monday. The nurse came in to give me all of my medicine one last time after the doctor came in to discharge me and give me my instructions. The nurse also went over the instructions and reminded me to make my appointment to see the doctor in a week to get the staples removed. I was ready to go home so I was very attentive to what was being said to me. It finally came time to depart the hospital and I was glad about that. The nurse rolled me down in the wheelchair while we waited for Elroy to bring the car around. It was really windy and cold outside but I didn't mind because I was going home.

Whenever I got home from the hospital, I had difficulty trying to walk up the stairs. I live in a townhouse and the kitchen and family room are on the second floor, so I had to walk up the stairs to get to that point. It seems that the sharp pain in my right leg was excruciating. I did manage to get to the third floor to lie down. The third floor is where the Master bedroom is and that is where I spent mostly all of my time. The pain kept shooting through my leg so intense that my husband had to call Dr. Koen. He immediately ordered a CT scan of my leg to rule out deep vein thrombosis which could have been a blood clot from the surgery. While in the ICU after surgery, I had a machine that was attached to my legs that pumped constantly to keep the blood flowing so I was quite astonished to be experiencing this type of pain. I had to go the next day for this test. My husband, daughter from Washington and her two kids accompanied me, agaain, for this test. We had to be there by 7:00 a.m. the next morning and believe me, I was not prepared to go any place after just being released the day before from the hospital with 37 staples in my head, but this was something that I had to do. I did not want to go back to the hospital with a blood clot because that could be very serious as well. I did have a surgical bonnet on my head to conceal the staples. This became my constant companion until the staples were removed. When visitors came to see me at home, I had the bonnet on and would take it off if they wanted to see the staples. I didn't mind because these were family and friends. It was something to see with all that metal in my head. Everybody that saw it asked me did it hurt. I would tell them that I didn't feel anything. I would stare at them in the mirror and wonder how they would heal and what impact would the scar have on my life. We, as women, are very serious about our appearances, so my curiosity was very strong until the staples would be removed and I could see the final results. I didn't have much longer to wait.

I had the procedure done, which wasn't that bad because my husband was there to assist me. I did not have to totally disrobe but had to take my outer clothes off from the waist down. The procedure took about 20 minutes and afterwards, my husband came in to help me get dressed and we were on our way back home.

We got the results the next day which revealed there were no blood clots and all the vessels were clear. We figured that it was just one of those things when you lay down for an extended period of time and don't use muscles, they can become taut and that is what happened to me. I was in the hospital for 3 days just laying down and only getting up to use the bathroom. I was pleased with those results because I knew I had a long road ahead from the surgery and didn't need any other obstacles or complications in my way. So, I endured the pain for a few more days and then suddenly it went away.

The surgeon had suggested that I shampoo my hair when I got home but this was not a good idea. My head was way too sore to accomplish this feat. My daughters went and bought some baby shampoo and tried but the pain was just too intense. So, they managed to get some of the blood out by pouring it on the hair and not rubbing too hard. That was a little successful but very messy. Needless to say, we didn't try that again.

As I recuperated at home, my husband was there every step of the way because my daughter had to leave to go back to Washington to be with her husband. He was missing her and I understood what he was going through. I was very happy that she was able to come to be with me before, during and at least a week after my surgery. Just to have the grand kids around made everything less painful because every morning, my grandson, Xavier, who was 4 at the time, would come upstairs to my room to ask me if I felt better. My eye was swollen shut after the surgery and after I got home. He would also ask me if I could open my eye to see him. Little did he know that I could always see him out of my left eye, so I would answer him that I could see him. He would look at me and see that eye was still shut, but he accepted my answer and then proceeded to play his Leapfrog game and explain different parts of the game to me. That was really special to me, too. He knew that his grammy was sick because he was at the hospital when I went in to have my surgery and my granddaughter, Adrianna, explained things to him the best that an 11 year old could do. They are great kids who I love very much and was thankful that I woke up to see them after I got home. They couldn't see me immediately after surgery because I was in ICU and they were not old enough to come in to see me. I understood the rules and regulations governing patients in ICU and as long as I knew they were okay, that made me feel good and determined to recover from this surgery. Whenever you have little ones that depend on you and really love you, it makes even the most painful surgery ever imaginable more tolerable. You can tolerate the excruciating pain just knowing that you have special ones praying for you and asking God to make the pain go away. That will surely keep you going. Trust me.

Chapter 6

The Healing and Recuperation Begins

The healing process was a slow process. If you look at the big picture, then you can see why it took a long time to go through this process. Remember, I had brain surgery. That is not something people have everyday. To be at home was bad and good. The pain in my head was very severe and I was on some pretty powerful pain medication and also steroids. It was an effort to just be able to take these medications during the day and night. The pain was the most severe early in the morning. The pain medicine made me feel like I was not myself because I was not able to get out of bed without feeling like I was going to fall. It was a scary feeling but I had my daughter and husband there with me to assist me to the bathroom and to make sure I had something to eat. I am a very independent person and some things I did for myself, but it wasn't an easy task most of the time, but I felt that I had to keep some of my independence if I could. That made me feel like I was going to get better to take care of myself, totally. Well, that didn't quite come to pass, because there was no way I could take care of myself at all for the first three weeks and was thankful that my husband had taken time off from work to be there with me. That was the best care that I could ask for during the first days at home for recuperation.

As days went by, I was basically bedridden for the first two weeks. Just to try to do normal and/or simple things were next to impossible. Whenever you can barely lift your head off the pillow and have to sleep always on the left side takes getting used to and you wonder how long will this last. I was asking myself this constantly and praying to God to make the pain go away. I keep talking about pain because there is a lot of it following this surgery. While in the hospital, you get medicines constantly to control the pain and the doctor prescribes that pain medicine in pill form which is supposed to work the same way as the medicine they put in your IV. The medicine in the IV is going directly into your blood stream at that particular time. When you take the pill, it has to dissolve and then start to work. It does work but not as fast. I didn't want to stay on those pain pills because they were habit forming and I did not want to be dependent on narcotics. My system did not agree with them because I had to take a nausea pill along with the pain pill. They literally made me sick to the point of vomiting. The doctor changed from those pills and prescribed another pain pill which was also a narcotic that made me sick to my stomach. I knew from those experiences that I would never be a drug user because I don't like how they make me feel and I don't like feeling nauseous. Needless to say, I was prescribed another pain medication that was not a narcotic but still made me nauseous. They help ease my pain and that is very good. I continue to take them, along with the nausea pill. This pain is so severe that all I could do was shed tears. It was hard for tears to stream from my right eye because it was still healing. It would open during the day but by the evening, it would just close on its own and I could not, for the life of me, make it open. When it wanted to reopen, it would on its own and that was a surprising experience. The nerves were ready to go to sleep and it made the eye ready for that process. When it was ready to wake up, it did. It's amazing what nerves in your body are capable of doing. They get their directions from the brain and my brain was probably working overtime trying to recover from the invasion of the tumor and the surgery. It had been through something for God knows how long.

CHAPTER 7

Elroy Jones, My Husband

He thought I was not going to make it. He said he was thinking, while I was in surgery, what would he do without me? That was a constant reminder during those long hours while he was waiting for the outcome. Those are the words that he revealed to me and I was glad that I made it to please him and to put those thoughts out of his mind.

Elroy Jones is my husband of 28 years. I thank God everyday for the care he provided to me from the first day of the news of the tumor (the ultimate surprise) until this day 8 months later. My illness has had a huge impact on our lives and finances, as well. He used all of his leave on his job to spend the first three weeks at home taking care of my every needs. He was my one and only caretaker at that time and I am very thankful for the care he provided and I want to thank him for being a part of my life and well-being. He was under stress with the day to day care of me and trying to survive and deal with the traumatic situation that caught us by surprise. This was totally unexpected. He was there to administer all of my medicine as well as prepare three meals a day (breakfast, lunch and dinner). We had several friends who provided food the first 2 weeks after surgery. That made things a little easier for him. He made sure I ate what I could and that all of my needs were met from taking baths to making sure I had clean pajamas to put on. He performed all tasks that needed to be done in the household. He would not leave my side except to go to the store. To this day, 8 months later, he still only goes to the store after we get home from work. Since I have not been able to drive during all of this time, he picks me up everyday and brings me home. After I get home, he makes sure that I get my rest by taking the phone off the hook so no one will call to disturb me because I really go to sleep everyday when I get home because of the fatigue.

The first two weeks were the most trying and difficult. He assisted me with going up and down the stairs, checking the incision to make sure there was no leakage and thankful there wasn't any. The staples kept everything in tact which he counted all 37 of them. He made sure that I took all the medicine that was prescribed as well as picking up the prescriptions from the pharmacy. When the pain struck in the middle of the night, he would jump up, go downstairs and get the pain medication. I was confined to the bed most of the day. When I would go downstairs, I would go back up in the early evening. I mostly had dinner in bed, as well as other meals for the first two weeks. I was able to see some friends for short periods of time during the first two weeks, also. Since I am diabetic, the steroids had my blood sugar elevated and I had to check it closely everyday. He was there to do that for me and to record the readings. We were both happy when the readings were normal once again.

One thing we missed this year was a vacation. I was going through my radiation treatments and was not feeling like doing anything but rest. Our anniversary is August 2nd and as I mentioned earlier, we have been married 28 years because we got married in 1980. We have always planned our vacations around our anniversary, so our hopes are that in 2009, we can start our tradition once again. Each and everyday we thank God that he made me a survivor and I have Elroy to spend my time with. He says that I am still incapacitated but with God's blessing we are able to strive everyday. He takes each day in stride because he knows we have the Lord on our side and without Him we could not make it or never would have made it. He is the reason for my survival after the surgery. These are words he believe in and try to live by each day.

During the summer months, we would usually grill out several times a week and that was something I couldn't do so he did it. He basically catered to my every need without any remorse or aggravation. He did this because he loves me unconditionally and he lives up to the vows we took 28 years ago before my father who performed our ceremony and God.

Elroy is one of the best husbands God created and I am the one who is very thankful for having him in my life. He admitted to me that he was very optimistic about the surgery and he prayed constantly while I was in that operating room. He said he wouldn't know what to do if he lost me because I complete him. He is very devoted to my every need, even today. He knows all of my limitations and always has a watchful eye on my every move.

During my recovery he had a part-time cleaning job for about 2 weeks in September. He had concerns about taking the job because he was worried about leaving me at home alone. I tried to reassure him that I would be alright even though I could not convince myself because I was not used to being by myself since the surgery. He felt like this was something that he had to do to help with the financial crunch we were facing due to my illness, so he went to work from about 6:00 p.m. until 10:00 p.m. He called at least every half hour every night that he was away from me. I mainly slept while he was away and did miss him, but I followed his instructions before he left and knew what to do and what not to do while he was away. I had finished my radiation treatments but was still feeling the side effects from them, so fatigue was the main side effect which made me really tired and all I needed was sleep and that is what I did until he came back home.

To date, he is very doting and knows when I am in pain and not feeling well. He can just look at me and my body language to tell me how I am feeling and most of the time he is one hundred percent correct. He is my confidante and a blessing from God Almighty. Whenever we are out shopping, he makes sure I hold onto him when we are walking so I won't fall because sometimes my balance is off and I stumble. I know everybody reading this might say that is what a husband is supposed to do; take care of his wife when she is sick (in sickness and health til death do you part). I agree with these assumptions, but I just feel that he has gone far beyond just being a husband. The Lord will truly bless him because he never wavered, quivered or mumbled anything negative since he's been taking care of me. I wouldn't want anybody else to take care of me but him. I show my appreciation by saying thank you with every plate of food he prepares for me, when he gives me the numerous pills I have to take and when I should take them, and for just loving me with no strings attached.

As I was writing this book, I could not think of a title, so I asked for his assistance. After pondering for a few minutes, he announced, "The Ultimate Surprise" and I asked him why that title and he said "simply because the Lord said that it was the ultimate surprise". That brain tumor was not expected and it took us all by surprise, so he felt that would be the best title and I agree with him.

Elroy is a vital part of my life and we were meant to be together. He would always say to me and everybody who asked about me that I'm not out of the woods yet. He still worries a lot and restricts what I can and can't do around the house. When I am able to do something, he would say "very good, little grasshopper" and that always makes me laugh. He says that he has to stay healthy to take care of me and so far he has done that. He's very lucky not to have any health issues at this time.

CHAPTER 8

Daughter Returns Home,
Sister & Parents Visit

The week after I came home, my daughter had to prepare for her trip back to Oak Harbor, Washington, but at least she was there when my sister and her daughter came to see me the Friday after I was released from the hospital. They just came up for the day to see exactly how I was doing since I was not in the hospital. I was in the bed on the third floor when they came and that is where I remained during their visit. My sister felt that I should have still been in the hospital but I had to reassure her that I was doing okay at home and Elroy was taking really, really good care of me. They were telling me how worried he was while I was in surgery and how he could finally breathe when the surgeon came out to say everything went well and I was doing alright. They could see his tender care while they were there because he never failed to come upstairs to check on me despite their presence. He felt that it was his duty to care for me and that is what he was doing. After she was completely satisfied with me doing okay, they had to make the trip back to North Carolina.

On Saturday, the next day, my mother (Bessie Laprade), her husband Lacey Laprade), my mother-in-law and father-in-law (Vertie & L.V. Jones) from North Carolina came to see me. They all came for a few hours to see exactly how I was doing for themselves. They all had sad faces when they saw the staples in my head. I was not in the bed on the third floor, but was in the family room on the second floor awaiting their visit. I told them that I did not feel the staples and that I was going to be alright. They were concerned about how I would feel when they would be removed, which was the next week.

I sort of reassured them that everything would be okay. I was not too convincing to them because my father-in-law had staples after one of his surgeries and he said they really hurt when they were removed. I sympathized with him, but still felt that this would be less painful. I told them that it can't hurt no more than the pain I feel in my head constantly from the surgery. I think that finally reassured them and I told them that Elroy would let them know how I did once they are removed. I hated to see them leave but I knew they had to make the three hour trip back before it got too late. I felt good after they left because it made me feel very special that they made the trip to Virginia just to see me.

Elroy's mother was very impressed with the way he was caring for me. She said she taught him how to do certain things (cleaning, cooking, laundry, etc.) so he would be able to do these things when he got married. She wanted him to be prepared to take care of his wife and take over the household duties while she was incapacitated. I thanked her for her teachings to him because he was doing an excellent job for this first week and she knew that he would continue to do this during my recuperation. My mother's mind was at ease, also, because she could see how he was taking care of me, too. I assured them that they did not have to worry about me as long as I had him here.

My daughter, Jacqueline, and grandsons are getting ready to leave. This is Sunday and I sure wish I could accompany them to the airport and see them get on the plane like I did in November when my daughter and grandson initially left to go to their new location in Oak Harbor, Washington, but that was not possible. It had only been one week since I've had the surgery and I've been home for seven days. I was very sad to see her and the children leave me but I knew she had her husband, who has been without her for 2 weeks, at home waiting for her, so I had to let go. The tears that came to my eyes as she and the boys were leaving were definitely not tears of joy. I was missing her and the kids already, but I had to stop and check myself because I could not let anything interfere with my healing process. It wasn't easy but it helped to talk about them and that made it worthwhile. Jameka, my oldest daughter, drove them to the airport and that was good because they had a chance to spend some sisterly and quality time together before she and the boys went to the gate to await their departure. That made me feel good because that is what sisters do for each other. I was happy that my two daughters were close and loved each other.

I was delighted to get the call that they made it home safely without any delays or problems. Traveling alone with two small kids, one being an infant, is not an easy task and I admire her for doing this for me. She was determined that she would be with me and that made me feel warm all over that she would do that for me. To travel that distance with small kids was remarkable to me.

CHAPTER 9

Staples Removed

My appointment with the surgeon was fast approaching and I was sort of dreading my visit to him because he would be removing the staples from my head. I am feeling both anticipation and anxiety as the day draws near. We go to his office and wait to be seen. Once in the examination room, we wait patiently for the surgeon to make his appearance. When he finally comes in, he immediately asks me how I am doing and then proceed to do some tests. The first test is the "follow my finger" test. This will let him know if I still have the double vision, which I did, and he was expecting me to still have it. He then proceeded to stick safety pins in my face, which I did not feel. That, too, would have been expected. Can you just imagine a doctor sticking pins in your face? It made you feel like you were a voo-doo doll. I hope I didn't bring anybody any bad luck! But I really didn't feel it, though. Just the thought of him doing that was sort of comical to us.

Now, it is time for the ultimate staple removal. I was very nervous as he pulled out his instrument, which was a special staple remover, and proceeded to perform this task. The first staple he removed bled and he was pleased that the blood flow was good. I was scared because I could feel the blood on my forehead which he generously wiped away. By the way, he started from the front and worked his way toward the back. He continued to remove each staple and there was no more blood and I did not feel anything. He was pleased with each removal and that built up his confidence to keep going. He finally told me to breathe. I did not realize that I wasn't breathing but apparently I wasn't. Remember, this doctor is pulling staples out of my head and I am on the frightened side, so if I wasn't breathing, I wasn't breathing. As he pulled the last staple out, he was pleased with how the incision looked and he praised me for being such a good patient. I asked the surgeon how long will it be before I fully recovered from this surgery. He said it could take up to one year for all of the nerves to be like they were before surgery and some nerves might not heal. I said one year is a long time. He agreed but that is the way it is. I was glad this appointment was over and wanted to know what do I do now. He told me to go home and continue to rest until I come see him again.

CHAPTER 10

Death of My Brother

As I was going through my healing process, I lost my oldest brother, Harry Patrick. He suffered a stroke in 2006 and his life was never the same again. He was not able to talk, communicate or recognize anybody. He was not improving and there was nothing the doctors in Richmond could do for him. He was constantly in and out of the hospital and was not getting any better. We were praying for a miracle so he could get better because today, people are surviving strokes at an alarming rate and we were hoping that he would be one of them, too. That wasn't going to happen. When he was released from the hospital, he was placed in a facility but he still was not improving. His daughter, Jennifer, took it upon herself to take him out of the facility and care for her father herself because the care he was receiving in the facility was less than tragic and she was not satisfied. My husband and I made several visits to see him when he was hospitalized as well as when he was in the facility. I felt I had to be there for Jennifer because she was going through a stressful time and needed my support which I was happy to give to her. These visits were made before I found out about my condition and my future, as well.

During my last visit to him, he was not doing too good and mainly just slept while we were there. I knew that things were not good for him and were not going to get better. A month before he died, the doctor placed him in hospice care and discontinued the feedings. This was when Jennifer called all of us together to visit with him. This gave my sisters and mother a chance to see him because they had not been to visit him during his illness and it was now or never. They all made the trip to see him and reminisced about our childhood. He was always a very humble person who never gave our parents any trouble. He would always work and spend his spare time at the Boys Club and out of harm's way. He was just a genuinely good person and father who cared for his daughters very much.

Since he had his stroke, he was not able to take any food or water orally because he could not swallow. All food and liquids were fed through a tube in his stomach. His body was rejecting the food and it was backing up in the tubes. This might seem unhuman for the doctor to order this, but that was the case. His body was shutting down and his daughter and the hospice team were there to make sure he was comfortable and clean. He couldn't do anything for himself. He was helpless. It was really sad to see someone you love in that condition. He didn't look like himself and my heart just went out to him as I wished he would recognize me. That didn't happen. It wasn't long after I made this visit that I found out about my condition and was unable to make any more visits to him.

On May 21, 2008, while I was still home recuperating, Jennifer called to tell me that my brother had just died. It was 3:00 p.m. and she was waiting for the Medical Examiner to pronounce him dead and the Mortician to come and pick him up. I was sad and hurt but I knew he was out of his misery because for 2 years he didn't have a life, he was just existing. When I would go and visit him, he did not recognize me at all. That hurt me just as much as him dying. For him not to recognize me when I went to visit him, I knew that he was just existing. He was my oldest brother and we grew up together. I loved him very much.

The funeral was held on May 27, the day after Memorial Day, and it was very difficult for me to make that trip because it had only been one month since I had my surgery and I was still recuperating myself but I had to go because that was my oldest brother and I had to be there for Jennifer. She needed our support. I did have a chance to see my sisters, brother and mother which made me feel good to see them again. Everybody was very helpful with me and made sure that I had my balance when I was walking, especially at the funeral. Elroy was a pallbearer which meant he could not be with me because they had to sit away from us, so my brother assisted me to my seat, sat with me and helped me to get back to the car after the funeral.

I was thankful that Elroy was able to take me to the funeral since this was a work day after a holiday. Some employers frown on employees taking an unplanned day off after a holiday, but this was an unforseen event that we didn't see coming at the time. He did not encounter any problems from his employer based on the circumstances for him not reporting to work. We were very thankful for that.

I think about my brother everyday but know that he is in God's hands and is not suffering anymore. I know he is in heaven. His death was very devastating to my mother because she was worried about me and my outcome and now she loses her oldest son. She said it is worse on a parent when they lose a child. I tried to reassure her that I am almost positive that I'll heal completely and not to worry about me. My prognosis and outlook were good and even though I am in this state now, it has only been one month since surgery. That put her mind at ease so she could concentrate just on the loss of one child. I understood her dilemma as a parent but did not want her to count me out yet. I still have some living and some healing to do so we got through this ordeal.

Chapter 11

Spiritual Awakening

On a special day during my recuperation, DeLaine Stieff, who came back into my life. At this particular time, I was home alone as Elroy had returned to work. Her purpose was to comfort me and to see how I was doing. As we were talking and communicating, she asked me if she could pray for me. Of course I said yes because she was a strong Christian woman who had amazing powers and vision from God.

As she began to pray, a warm feeling overcame me that I never felt or experienced before. The more she prayed, the warmer I felt. This was a spiritual awakening that I am sure assisted in the healing process. I started to cry and the tears overflowed and wouldn't stop. The power of prayer and the presence of God was overwhelming. As she finished the prayer, we sat and waited for the tears to finally stop flowing. As the visit came to an end, she wrote this verse for me to say each day for the remainder of my recovery:

Thank you for my healing:
I think about His love and
I think about His goodness.
I think about His grace
That has brought me through.
For as high as the heavens above
So great is the measure of my Father's love;
Great is the measure of my Father's love.
Thank you for healing me!

She is truly a strong Christian friend and I am thankful that she is my dear friend; more like a sister. She uplifted my spirit and made me feel good about myself. It is a wonderful feeling that when you are sick, all friends come to your aid and offer assistance to you when you need it. She did that for me and I am forever grateful for her. To have a close relationship with God is truly remarkable and to spread His word to others is gracious.

DeLaine came back into my life and showed me spiritual support, transportation assistance and financial support. I was very blessed that she came back into my life at this particular time and I can never thank her enough for her generosity and sisterly love. It was very much appreciated.

CHAPTER 12

Return to Work

I felt that it was time for me to return to work. My surgeon didn't quite agree with me but I convinced him that this was something that I felt like I could do and needed to do for myself. He felt that I should stay out for at least three months, but I knew it was not going to take that long for me to return to work. On June 2, 2008, I went to work. After the funeral of my brother and being surrounded by family, the time was right. Trust me, I was the only one who felt that I should return to work. I knew that driving was out of the question because of the double vision but I had a plan. My daughter was still here, so she was my driver during my first few days. I was only allowed to work 4 hours a day, so I had to get off at 12:00 noon. This proved to be a challenge because even though my daughter had some flexibility at work, it was not always possible for her to be at my beck and call everyday at noon. My husband couldn't be there at 12:00 to pick me up because he was basically just returning back to work himself and his leave was exhausted. So, my dilemma was getting ready to start and I did not know exactly what I was going to do at this time. I knew I wanted to keep going to work, but my transportation was not quite worked out before I made that decision. I had to get my brain working for sure to get through this pitfall.

That is where my co-workers and neighbor stepped in and offered assistance. By noon, I was ready to go home because at this time, I was still in a lot of pain, my vision wasn't good and my balance was even worse. I was able to get back in the work mode and do whatever task that was presented to me but I had to be careful and always watch my steps. I couldn't just jump out of my seat and start moving. I had to gently arise, get my bearings and proceed to walk.

If I didn't do it quite right, I knew I would end up on the floor and that was a chance I was not willing to take. If I ended on the floor, I knew I would end up back home recuperating for more weeks.

To be back at work made me feel extra good about myself because I was still able to comprehend and accomplish different tasks. I am convinced that once you have a brain tumor and have it removed, people seem to think that a part of your senses left with the removal of that tumor. I proved otherwise because it seems my mind was sharper than before. I could still remember everything I needed to remember and some things I had forgotten about over the years. That is a blessing to come through that type of surgery all in tact and in one piece.

I got through my days at work and looked forward to each day that I was there. I love my job and that is nothing new. I looked forward to coming to work before the ultimate surprise took over my life. It was difficult, but with the support of my bosses and some of my co-workers, it was all good. They were there for me when I really was feeling my worse and they were very sympathetic when I talked to them about how the pain was trying to take over. It didn't quite have that much power because I was able to medicate myself to ease the pain and keep working. My job is not a stressful one as long as I can do it. I am a diligent worker and very meticulous in the finished product so I couldn't let something like pain deter me from completing my work. I was back on the job to do what was expected from me and that is what I did without any special privileges. To me, my job is very important because I work for the two top bosses and my work reflects on them. I don't want anything negative to have any effects on them or the Airport Authority®. They have too many years invested in the day-to-day operation of the airport and that is very essential to its success.

Diane stepped in to take me home. I really didn't want her to do this because she is the receptionist and her job is very important. She took her lunch hour to take me home and some leave time because she couldn't get back in time. She was adamant about doing this and I didn't give her much argument because I just wanted to get home. I was glad when my neighbor, Amanda, stepped in when she did. That solved a lot of problems for me.

As I was getting better, my doctor increased my work days, again, at my request. He listens to me and if I tell him I think I can do something, he lets me do it. The longer days were very tiring at first. When your body gets used to one thing, it has to adjust to something else. I had gotten used to being home and asleep by 1:30 p.m. and now I was working until 3:00 p.m. every day. By 1:30 p.m., I was very drowsy and sleepy. It was not difficult for me to take a power nap at 1:30 p.m., because technically, I was at lunch from 1:00-2:00 even though I didn't eat everyday, I was able to rest for a part of that hour. As the days progressed, the drowsiness subsided until I got home around 3:30 p.m. and I was able to rest at 4:00 p.m. That worked very well and, again, my body got used to that time.

As I move into the next chapter, the 4:00 time became 4:30 and that is what it still is today.

CHAPTER 13

Radiation Therapy

My surgeon had informed me earlier after surgery that I would need radiation treatments to try to kill the cells that were left from the tumor. The cells are in my sinus cavity that is surrounded by blood vessels and nerves that, during the surgery, he didn't want to disturb because it could leave me speech impaired and/or paralyzed. I was glad that he chose that option because those are conditions that I did not want to endure for the rest of my life.

He made me an appointment to see an Oncologist who will oversee and administer the radiation treatments. He is specialized in chemotherapy and radiation. My first appointment with him was a consultation appointment. The nurse took my vitals and asked me questions regarding my medical history. After she finished, the doctor came in and reviewed my medical history, went over the X-rays and explained the treatment course as well as potential side effects. He explained that there were two options they were considering for the cells. The first option was an all day treatment in the hospital with my head anchored down while the rays were administered. That sort of scared me and I really didn't want that option. The second option was a 5 week, 5 days a week treatment regiment. This sounded better but I was concerned with transportation. He further explained that he would be meeting with my surgeon and other team members to go over my record. He also explained that I would have to have a CT scan so he will have a module to go by as he targets the tumor. He told me there were two cells that they must try to destroy. Since it is a slow growing tumor it is best to radiate it during the 5 week period. He said they wanted to be careful when administering the radiation and not interfere with heathy cells in the process. Accuracy in the rays was very essential and vital for the success in the treatment.

Before I actually began treatment, there was some technical planning with a specialized CT machine in order to pinpoint the exact areas that needed to be treated. The process is called Simulation and it is the preparatory phase prior to the treatment and would last approximately one hour. Simulation is done on a machine that is very similar to the machine on which the treatments are done. The Radiation Therapist scanned the head. After the simulation, the physician identified the exact areas that need the radiation as well as the area that would need protection from the rays.

The CT scan was scheduled and I had it done. I now must have a mask made to fit my face so the markings can be on it for the duration of the radiation treatments. This was an experience because I still had some swelling and pain but I knew this was a requirement since they couldn't put the markings on my right temple because it would wash away when I washed my face. Well, we got the mask made and now it was time to schedule my appointments. I met again with the nurse and she provided me with several pamphlets on cancer which was very disturbing to me. The surgeon, as well as the Oncologist, have assured me more than once that my tumor was not cancerous yet I get all of this information on cancer. She told me what to expect from the radiation. One thing was hair loss in the treatment area. When I was told this, I went to my beautician, Nikki, and told her what the nurse told me. She gave me a cute hair cut that got me lots of compliments. Everybody was telling me that I looked much younger with the short hair. Hearing those remarks made me feel even more positive about myself and I felt I can conquer these radiation treatments. Ronnikka Williams (Nikki) said that if I did lose hair, it wouldn't be as noticeable since my hair would already be short. Needless to say, I didn't lose much hair. What I lost was like the nurse advised; in the treatment area and you couldn't tell because I still had hair to cover it based on the haircut I received from Nikki. Thank you Nikki for taking care of me these past six years. She is like my third daughter.

Also, with the hair, I couldn't use any harsh shampoo or any chemicals on my hair. I could only use a blow dryer with mild heat. During my treatment, hair washes were few because it was still painful and I didn't feel like going to the hair salon. I did okay with the few washes and again, didn't lose too much hair. I did notice that when I combed my hair, there was a lot in the comb but I didn't panic because I knew this would happen. I just kept combing and destroying the hair that was in the comb. After the treatments were completed, I went to the salon and felt good after I left because I knew my hair was clean and once again, Nikki did an outstanding job and I was a happy customer.

The main side effect that affected me during the radiation treatments the most was fatigue. I was told that if I felt tired, I should rest and that is what I did. I was working 6 hours a day and when I left work to go to treatments, I was already tired. After treatment, when I went home, I immediately went to sleep for at least two hours. It was needed and my body was telling me to rest. I had no control over this fatigue; it had control over me and all I could do was give in and rest. It has been three months since radiation and I still have to rest when I get home from work.

Other side affects is loss of appetite and she advised that I should not lose any weight while going through treatments. If this should happen, I would have to meet with a Nutritionist. I was able to maintain my weight and that was not a problem for me. Even though I didn't lose any weight, I managed not to gain any. I watched what I ate and tried to be as careful as possible.

Another side effect is very dry skin and I am still dealing with that several months after treatment. I am still searching for the perfect remedy to rid my skin of this dryness. I shall keep looking until I find it. If not, I will seek the assistance of a Dermatologist. My face is the worst and I keep lotion on it so the flakiness won't come through. The right side is discolored and I am waiting for the skin tone to be even again.

The special care instructions for radiation treatments to the brain were:

1. Please make sure you do not wash off your marks. Gently cleanse the hair with a mild shampoo such as baby shampoo and be careful not to rub marks off. Gently pat hair with a towel. (I did not have any marks because I had the mask. I used the baby shampoo when I washed my hair myself).

2. *DO NOT* use any harsh shampoos, hair dryers or hair setting solutions. (I didn't use any harsh shampoos, but did use the blow dryer. The nurse advised that I could as long as it was on a low setting. That worked fine for me).

3. The skin in the treatment area may **become red, dry, and itchy.** Your hair may fall out but will re-grow in time. The skin the treatment area may **become red, dry and itchy.** *DO NOT* use any lotion, oil, powders, creams, perfumes, or soaps, in the treatment area other that what the nurse or doctor recommends. (My hair loss in the treatment area was minimal and I followed these instructions very carefully).

4. *DO NOT* expose the treatment area to direct sunlight. After completing all treatments, use a SPF 15 or greater sunscreen on the treatment area when out in the direct sunlight, and wear a wide brimmed hat. (I was not exposed to direct sunlight much and mainly stayed inside away from the sun. I did notice that when I was in the sun when I was out shopping, the sun did emit a burning sensation, so I immediately went inside until the sun set).

5. *DO NOT* use hot water bottles, heating pads, or ice packs on the treatment area.
(I adhered to this instruction and did not have a use for either of these).

6. If taking steroids, maintain your schedule daily as directed by your doctor. *Never abruptly stop taking steroids.* (I was taking steroids and did abruptly stop taking them because my insurance would not refill them. I initially was taking one-half pill a day but the doctor changed the dosage to one pill a day which made me use them sooner than the prescribed dosage.

I didn't have another choice but to not get them refilled. That was a dilemma that I had no control over, so, therefore, that was the end of my taking the steroids. I didn't feel any different by not taking them)

7. Please report any headaches, nausea, vomiting, visual changes, seizure, and weakness in the arms or legs. (The only thing I reported was the headaches, which I still had daily from the surgery. I continued to take my medications before going to treatment which made it less painful during the procedures. I did not have any of the other affects).

8. It is important to maintain a well-balanced diet, adequate fluid intake, and a stable weight throughout treatment. (Tell your nurse, doctor or therapist, if you are having nausea or diarrhea). (I was able to maintain a stable weight throughout treatment and did not experience any nausea or diarrhea. As a matter of fact, I was taking medication for nausea that was a side affect from my pain medication, so I was protected from the nausea).

9. Your energy level and sleeping patterns may change as your body works hard to repair itself. If you feel tired during treatment, rest and relaxation can help your body recover. Expect to stop feeling fatigued a few weeks after your treatment end. (This is very true. The fatigue was relevant while I was going through treatment and it is still that way today. My body tells me when I need to rest and I give in every time. Fatigue is something that has to be dealt with because you just can't function when you are tired. Each and everyday when I came from treatment, I went to sleep. I was never a person who would sleep a lot because I tried to stay active, but this is something that you have to give into and that is what I did. It made me feel better after I rested).

10. You will visit your physician at least once per week during your treatment. Blood pressure, temperature, weight and blood work may be obtained at this time. (Doctor day was Wednesday of each week, or if you were having any special

problems, a doctor was always available. That was a plus and I has some issues before doctor day and was able to see the doctor. I looked forward to seeing the doctor every week because he would listen to me and really cared about how I was feeling. He would tell me that I was tolerating the treatments very good and that was a plus).

11. Treatments are given Monday through Friday. No treatments are given on weekends or holidays. The total number of treatments you will receive will tentatively be 30. (I received the 30 treatments. I started treatment on July 17 and concluded the last treatment on September 2. The last treatment was supposed to be August 30, but that day the machines were not working, so I had to go through the Labor Day holiday and received the treatment the Tuesday after the holiday).

These are the instructions that were given to me by the Oncology Department.

More treatment instructions were:

- Radiation treatments are given daily Monday through Friday at the *same time each day*. The treatment itself only takes a few minutes, but your appointment is generally scheduled for 15-30 minutes, including allowance for set up time. The staff will work with you to try to schedule your daily appointment at a time that is convenient for you. When you enter the department for each of your radiation treatments that you sign in at the front desk. This allows the receptionist to know when you are there so she can then announce your arrival to the therapists on the treatment machine. At the first visit, a Radiation Therapist will greet you in the lobby and take you to the treatment area.

- You will be taken into the treatment room where, you will be asked to lie very still on the table. The staff will use the marks on your skin or the special masks to identify the treatment area. On your first visit and weekly thereafter, the staff will take X-rays to ensure the accuracy of your treatments. These

X-rays are for accuracy purposes only and will not provide the physician with any diagnostic information concerning how your cancer is responding. The Radiation therapists may put special blocks or shields between the machine and you. The physicians order such devices to block or protect the healthy tissue from the radiation.

- As the therapists prepare you for your treatments, you may see lights in the room, which are used to help align the treatment field. At the same time, the therapists may be moving the machine around your body. You may hear noises as the machine moves, but just remember that this is normal. The radiation therapists will need to leave the room while your treatments are being given, but you are not alone during this time. You are in constant view on a television screen and can be heard and talked to at all times for a microphone within the room. You will not see nor hear the radiation being given and most likely will not feel a thing. If you are concerned with anything that happens in the treatment room, ask the therapists to explain. After the treatments are given, you can continue with your day as planned, as the radiation will not affect your ability to think, to drive or to walk.

After I got my treatment schedule for the next 6 weeks which at first the Oncologist said it would be 5 weeks, 5 days a week for a total of 25 treatments. After the team met, they changed the treatments to 6 weeks, 5 days a week, for a total of 30 treatments. This was very unexpected and I was wondering how I was going to find transportation for an additional week of treatments. The schedule I initially received was to start July 17 at 11:40 a.m. The Oncology Nurse immediately contacted a volunteer organization to see if she could schedule transportation to and from treatments. Needless to say that didn't happen. The dilemma was that I worked in Norfolk and the treatment center was in Virginia Beach, which was too costly with the price of gas at the time and the use of volunteers. This was devastating because I felt like I was being punished because I was trying to work while dealing with the upcoming 30 radiation treatments. I also felt that I wasn't important enough because I did not have cancer. These were the feelings I was experiencing at the time. I have true respect for this organization that works closely with cancer patients but was very disappointed that they could not help me. When Plan A doesn't work, you go to Plan B and that is what I did. I knew I had to get to those appointments because they did not want you to miss any. It would delay the treatment plan they had for you and I didn't want that to happen.

With these first treatments at 11:40, I had my co-worker, Debbie, who so graciously used her lunch hour and leave time to take me and bring me back to work. I really didn't want her to keep doing this. She went back to work and asked other co-workers if they would assist and everyone that could help, offered their assistance. Before Debbie provided assistance, Gale, whose mother Diane, works with me provided several trips to and from treatment for me. I really appreciated her generosity because she had to come from Chesapeake to Norfolk to Virginia Beach and back to Norfolk everyday to take me. My friend, Jeanne, who is retired, provided some of the transportation for me to keep my other friends from taking off.

I felt that this was going nowhere with the time and transportation dilemma. I talked to the technician to see if she could change my appointments to the end of the day. That way I would have to only get transportation there and my husband would be able to pick me up when he got off work. That way, he wouldn't have to take leave and by the time he arrived at the treatment center, I would be finished and we could just go home. The treatment center is about 10-15 minutes from where we lived. The technician was able to give me a 4:00 p.m. time and that worked out perfectly.

With the 4:00 p.m. treatment time, I sent an email to my best friends asking for their assistance in providing a one-way trip to my treatments. After I sent out the email, it seems that as soon as I hit the "send" button, the emails started flowing. In a matter of approximately 30 minutes, I had my transportation problem solved. It was amazing how quickly these ladies responded. They told me that they had been waiting for me to ask for anything I needed and they were there to provide whatever I needed. Well, at this time I just needed rides to my treatments from the airport in Norfolk to

Virginia Beach. We made a schedule and let everybody know who had what day and the ones that didn't get a chance to assist were on standby in case of any unforseen circumstances from the drivers. Everything worked out really well and I had a chance to see friends who I had not seen since the surgery. This was truly a blessing to have these friends and I thank God for them everyday.

The treatments were going good with the exception of the fatigue and the swelling I was still experiencing as well as the pain in my head. The Oncologist prescribed a mild dosage of steroids to make the swelling subside. It worked to some degree. I know when there is swelling because after treatment, my husband would see me and call me Waffle Face. That meant that the mask was so tight that it made my face look like a waffle. I didn't like that but there wasn't anything I could do. The treatments were needed everyday so I had to deal with any discomfort that came my way.

With the treatment schedule, on Mondays, they took pictures so that made the treatment time a little longer because the pictures were taken before treatment. Wednesdays, were doctor day. This is the day that you actually see the doctor and he goes over the progress of the treatments. He could not tell whether or not the tumor is shrinking because an MRI had not been done. The MRI would have to come 3 months after the last treatment. I really don't think I should wait that long, but that's the way things are and I have to live with it. Fridays was the day to make sure all the rays are aligned right and they are hitting the marks on the mask. They never told me any findings or anything. I was just there to receive the treatments. The staff was very nice and catered to my every need if I had one. They are well suited for the job they have to do and can deal with all patients going through radiation as well as chemotherapy treatments. Some of the staff's lives had been touched by cancer in their families and in their lives, as well. I was blessed to have them care for me.

The instructions for Follow-up after Radiation Treatments were as follows:

- Once you have completed your treatments, you will be given a follow up appointment with your physician. The purpose of this visit is to see how you are doing after your radiation. If at any time you need to talk to us before your follow up visit, just call the department. The first appointment is usually in one month and less frequently thereafter. Certain diagnostic studies such as lab and X-ray tests may be ordered at this time. The follow-up visits normally take 45 minutes but possibly longer if testing is required. Your follow-up visits are important to us and we will work with you to find a time that is convenient for you.

- Should you have any questions or concerns, please do not hesitate to call.

Since I've been through all of the treatments, I still experience a burning sensation inside my body two months after the last treatment. I sit and wonder where all of that radiation goes after it hit the spot.

CHAPTER 14

Ear Infection During Treatment

During the last two weeks of treatment I contracted an ear infection in my right ear which is the side I was receiving the radiation treatments. This was the strangest feeling I had ever experienced. I woke up one morning and thought I was getting a sinus infection because it just felt weird with my ear and during my life, I've had several sinus infections. Every time I chewed, my right ear felt like it was filling up with something and I was having trouble with my hearing out of that ear. I then started experiencing pain in my right ear that was totally unbearable. When I went for my treatment, I mentioned this to my technician and she said she would contact the doctor so he could see me after treatment. After I finished my treatment, I went to see the doctor and explained my symptoms to him, he immediately looked inside my ear and could see the fluid in there. I asked him if this was from the radiation treatments and he said he didn't think so. He said he would make an appointment for me to see an ENT that was located in that building. I thanked him and left.

The first appointment with the ENT was a consultation and examination appointment. The doctor felt that I would need a hearing test from the Audiologist that was in his office. He saw the amount of fluid behind the ear drum and explained to me that it was a caramel color which meant that it was not infected. He went on to say that he would put a tube in that ear to help the fluid drain. I had heard of tubes being in children's ears but did not know it was an option for an adult. He asked the appointment secretary to make an appointment for early the next week for me to have the procedure.

When I went for the appointment to have the procedure, I had to first have the hearing test. I had never had a hearing test before. I went inside a booth and the Audiologist performed several tests. I don't think I had much hearing loss but there were some things that I could not hear clearly while in the booth. When that part of my appointment was completed, I went into the examination room where the procedure would be performed. I sat in a chair and when the doctor came in, I was laid all the way back in the chair and he did what he had to do. I didn't have much discomfort because he numbed the inside of my ear. He did inform me when he was getting ready to slice my eardrum. I felt some pain, but I didn't feel that much. The procedure took about 10 minutes. He gave me some antibiotic ear drops to use for 5 days so there would be no infection. That was the end of that procedure and I left after making an appointment for follow up in 2 weeks and went home to recuperate so I could go to work the next day.

After getting the ear drum punctured, I was still having problems and pain within the ear and the left ear was filling up and causing me pain, too. So, I called the doctor and he wanted to see me again. He checked the left ear and decided not to do anything to it. He asked me if it was popping and I told him that it was, so he said that as long it would pop, he would not bother it. He felt that it would eventually heal itself. He checked the right ear and said the hole was still in the eardrum but it was draining real good and to his satisfaction. I made an appointment to go back, hopefully for the last time.

One funny thing I can say about my first visit to the ENT. He asked me if I could slide my wig back so he could see my incision. I guess he felt that since I was going through radiation treatments, one of the side effects is hair loss and he figured that was what I had. I laughed and told him that I was not wearing a wig and I was thankful that I didn't lose my hair. I think he was embarrassed but I let him see my scar by peeling through my hair to find it. After he saw it, he asked me how did I know that I had a tumor. I explained that I didn't know. I started by telling him that I woke up one Saturday morning with an excruciating headache and knew something was wrong, but in my wildest dreams I never would have thought it was a tumor. We talked further about what I had went through and he was amazed that I looked as good as I did after going through something as traumatic as that. It is amazing to see the sympathetic look on everybody's face when I tell them about my brain tumor (the ultimate surprise).

I went to see the ENT for the last time. He examined both ears. The right ear had a scab on the eardrum which he said would eventually go away. The left ear was completely clear and he released me and told me to come see him if and when I had any other problems. That was the end of treatment with the ENT. Maybe not the end because the fullness is returning in the right ear but there is no pain associated with it at this time. I will wait until my doctor's visit with the surgeon to know what next steps to take. Hopefully, it will just go away and never come back.

Well, there is a problem with the right ear again. The fullness when I chew and when I go up and down the stairs. There is no pain but discomfort. I will wait until I see Dr. Koen and see what he says.

CHAPTER 15

Time To Shine Party

Jeanne & Fred Earley (very dear friends of mine) put together a "Jackie's Time To Shine Party" to celebrate the end of Radiation Treatments. The "Time to Shine" theme was Jeanne's idea because most people probably think you are radioactive after these treatments and emit a shiny glow as you enter the room. There were special friends in attendance at this intimate affair. I was very excited to see these friends and be in their presence. I could hardly wait for the time to come for Elroy and I to leave to go to Jeanne's house. I was so excited for this event that I did not want to take any pain medicine because I felt I would be sluggish and not able to enjoy my friends. Bad mistake! My watchful husband always kept his eyes on me and knew exactly when I was in pain and not feeling well. Until those pains, I was really having a wonderful time. As gatherings go, the ladies retreat to one area and the guys retreat to another, except for Wade. He is Laura's significant other who just like hanging out with the ladies. That was very different for us because how could we bash guys, when we had one in our presence? We enjoyed his company and therefore, did not bash any guys. But as the saying goes, all things must come to an end and when Elroy came to me, that was it. I was ready to go, but hated to leave good company. These ladies even brought gifts which I was not expecting. They had done so much for me already and still to come bearing gifts were truly amazing. This was an intimate party and I want to thank Jeanne and Fred for their hospitality as well as Charlie and Debbie Meads, Laura Barnes and Wade, Bonnie & Rob Sampere, John and Janet Rial and Susan Bates and Brian. Thank you and I appreciated everything you did for me when it was my time to shine.

CHAPTER 16

Doctor's Visit

Whenever I found out about the tumor, I was experiencing double vision. After surgery, the double vision was still there. One reason was the tumor was sitting on Nerve 6, which is the optic nerve. I went to my surgeon in September and at first when he saw me he was amazed at how good I looked. We discussed the radiation treatments since I was finished with them. He informed me that I would need an MRI in December since that would be 3 months after the last treatment. His office will set that up for me. Now it was time for him to see how I was really doing. He did the finger test where I have to follow his finger with my eyes. This was done to see if the double vision had improved. I knew it was improved because I had noticed for about 2 weeks that the double vision was subsiding. When he did the test, I informed him that I only saw one finger. He was amazed at that response and did the test again, and again, I saw one finger. We were both convinced that the double vision had gone away after 6 months since its onset. We were happy with these results. He did another test with a feather towards my right eye. I blinked really fast from that feather on my eye. I think that was to check my reflex and I passed that test, too. I asked him about the pain I am still experiencing. He reminded me that the pain is coming from the craniotomy. I asked him what was a craniotomy. He explained that anytime you have brain surgery, a craniotomy is performed when they have to go into your skull to reach the tumor. With my craniotomy, some of the bone broke and they had to use cement to put the bone back together. That is where the pain is coming from and it will take more time for it to heal on the inside. There are three titanium screws in my head, also. I'm not sure if I am having any effects from those. After all tests and examinations were completed, he said he wanted to see me in 3 months after I have the MRI. Well, the MRI is scheduled for December 1 and my appointment with him is December 8. We'll wait and see what the outcome is and that will lead to the final chapter in this book.

CHAPTER 17

Nerve Pain in Face

For about 2 weeks when I try to chew on my right side, I will get a burning sensation like someone was standing there holding a match to my face. When I drink or eat something cold, it felt like cool water running inside my jaw. I didn't know what was going on so I just dealt with it. On the weekend of November 8, I was with my family in North Carolina for a gathering when it was so unbearable, I was crying and ran out of the room. Now you know Elroy was right behind me reassuring me that I should not eat on the right side. I told him that I was eating on the left side and it was really burning like fire. My family was very concerned with what was going on but they knew Elroy would know what to do. It didn't get any better so on Monday, I called the surgeon's office and explained to the nurse what I was going through. I had to leave this information on her voice mail and wait for her to call me back. I waited all day while I was at work. I wouldn't leave my desk unless I had to go to the restroom. I didn't eat lunch because I couldn't eat. Diane brought me a strawberry frappuchina that was cold and I could drink it through a straw. It was time for me to leave to go home without hearing from the doctor. Elroy came to pick me up and we went by the doctor's office which was closed. It was only 4:30 and they were closed. As I was going home, I called my office to check my voice mail and there were no messages. I immediately called the doctor's office again and left a very distraught message because I was still in pain and needed some relief. I informed her that if I didn't hear from the doctor, I would seek medical attention from either the Urgent Care Center or another doctor. The next morning the doctor's office called me at home because it was the Veterans Day holiday and I was off that day. She asked if I had received her message. She had just received my message from yesterday and was very apologetic with not getting back with me earlier. She informed me that the doctor said the sensations that I was experiencing was from the nerves in my face. He had prescribed some medicine to alleviate the pain and sensations and had called it into my pharmacy they had on record. I informed her that I still use that pharmacy and thanked her. After I finished talking to her, I called my voice mail and listened to the message. Well, the message was from my doctor's office that was left at 5:10 p.m. which was after I had left at 4:00 and after the office closed at 5:00 and the message said exactly what she told me. I went to pick up the prescription and immediately took a dosage. I had some of the few side affects but after a week, I started feeling better. The side affects were dizziness and drowsiness that later subsided as I kept taking the medication. One thing about this medicine is these are huge orange capsules that seem to go down sideways and always get caught in my throat. I luckily always have something to eat at the time I take these capsules and that helps tremendously. I am hoping that I am coming to the end of the road to recovery. It has been a long road with lots of pain and obstacles. I have been able to control the pain with medication and we are still facing obstacles but we keep praying to God to make these obstacles go away and we know that He will do that for us. As I am finishing this book, my right ear is getting that full feeling again. I think I am catching a cold because I also have the sniffles. Let's hope this go away really fast and I can enjoy the upcoming holiday season. I can only pray that this will be short lived and will not cause me any problems.

I am happy that the huge orange capsules worked, but as a medication work for one ailment, there are side affects that cause problems to other areas of the body. That was the case with these capsules.

CHAPTER 18

MRI

Today is December 1st and I have to have the MRI done to see if any of the tumor is still present. We have been praying that it is all gone but this is the ultimate test. I will have to wait until December 8th to get the results once I see the doctor. I am sure I will have to get the film to take to him even though he will get a written report probably within a day or two after it has been completed.

Whenever I arrived at the Advanced Imaging Center, it was amazing that all paperwork for the MRI was there and I didn't have to do anything because I was pre-registered and the doctor had sent the necessary script to them. I did have to fill out the necessary medical form which I had to list the numerous medications that I take daily. Also, I had to check all medical conditions that I currently have which is high blood pressure and diabetes. By the time I filled out this time consuming form, I was called in for a lab. This was something totally new to me and the nurse stated that they get blood from all diabetics to check the creatnin level in the kidneys. This is needed to confirm whether or not the contrast could be administered to complete the MRI. I was happy that my kidney functions were normal and the contrast was administered.

The doctor had requested on his script that the films be given to me after the MRI and the technician gave me a copy to take to him when I have my appointment on December 8. I have to wait a full week before I know the results. I can wait because I am still praying that the radiation treatments worked miraculously,

CHAPTER 19

Doctor's Visit to Discuss MRI

The date and day had finally arrived for my visit to Dr. Koen to get the results of the MRI taken one week ago. With film in hand, Elroy and I arrived for my appointment only to find that appointments were running one hour behind. My appointment was scheduled for 1:30 p.m., so I knew that I would not be seen until at least 2:30 p.m. When I was finally called back to the examination room, I had lots of butterflies in my stomach and said lots of prayers. After waiting another 20 minutes in the examination room awaiting the arrival of Dr. Koen, he finally appeared with another doctor. I asked him if it was all gone and he immediately clarified that he did not tell me that it would be gone. He further stated that the radiation was still working and would be working at least for another 3 months. I asked him how could that be when I stopped radiation treatments 3 months ago. He explained that even though the treatments stopped 3 months ago, the radiation will keep working for 6 months, so to date, it is still working. He said the tumor is deteriorating but doing so slowly. He could tell by the film that it is shrinking. He went on to explain that the tumor was wrapped around so many nerves that it took longer to remove it. I asked him about the numbness I am still experiencing after 7 months and he said that the Neurontin that he prescribed should help alleviate some of the numbness and pain but it will just take time. He was explaining certain aspects of the surgery to the other doctor in medical terms which I didn't understand. I did recognize the sixth nerve he mentioned because I had heard that term several times through my follow-up visits. He checked the incision. I explained to him that it was still very tender to the touch especially when I tried to comb my hair. I asked him how long will I keep feeling these discomforts from the incision and the craniotomy. He said it could take up to 2 years to completely heal. I reminded him that he has always said one year, now it's moved to 2 years? He said with the reconstruction, yes, it could take up to 2 years.

The visit was coming to an end when I informed him of my book and what it was about. I asked if I could use his name in the book and if he would be willing to sign a waiver to that effect. He informed me that I could use his name and he would sign whatever he needed to sign. I think he was impressed that one of his patients was able to do this.

At the end of the visit, he informed me that he would need to see me in 6 months, June 2009. He also informed me that he would prefer that I continue to work 6 hours a day until I felt that I could work full-time. I will wait to see how this goes as we go into 2009.

I had a lot of anxious family and friends waiting to hear the outcome of this visit and I knew I had lots of calls to make. I managed to make most of the calls to everybody's satisfaction. I am sure it was not the news we all were anticipating, but nonetheless, ti was not another ultimate surprise. I am certain that this ultimate surprise will soon go completely away and leave us alone. We need to go on with our lives without this surprise hanging around.

I did mention to Dr. Koen about my ear and he suggested that I contact the ENT so he can check it out again. I decided to wait until after the holidays to do this since it was not hurting. With the holidays fast approaching, I just wanted to be doctor-free so I can enjoy the season and that is what I did.

CHAPTER 20

Family

This chapter is dedicated to the foundation of my life; my family. I am from a family of six children. We were raised in a two-parent home until I was 20 years old when my mother and father separated. I was the oldest child at home when my mother left my brother and sister with our father in 1972. As I reflect on those years, I was left to basically take care of my father, sister and brother which I did not hesitate to do because my father needed that care. He was a brick mason by trade and worked very hard to provide for us. Today, we truly believe that since my father and older brother have departed this life, they are now in Heaven watching over us. This might sound strange to some, but we, as a family, sincerely believe this.

We just held our Family Christmas Party on Saturday, December 20, 2008 with my 3 sisters (Shirley, Patricia and Dorothy), my mother and brother (Thomas), along with our spouses, children and grand-children. In my mother's case, great-grandchildren. I had one great niece and 2 great nephews I had never seen and it was a joy to finally see and meet them. What a wonderful festive time we had. My nephew Stevie Cox and his wife, Linda, opened their home to all of us and my niece, Sharonda Whitfield, prepared a most festive Christmas dinner. Her mother, (my oldest sister) Shirley Peacock assisted with some of the preparation. Stevie and Linda converted their garage to a first-class elegant dining hall equipped with round tables, gold linen tablecloths and buffet tables befitting such an occasion. We were all taken aback when we went to the garage because it was just like walking into a 4-star restaurant without the waiters. The weather was mild, so it was very comfortable temperature-wise. The atmosphere was also very amazing. Even though we were celebrating the togetherness of family, my brother-in-law, Rudolph Peacock, was celebrating his birthday, so we acknowledged this special day to him by singing Happy Birthday. He was very pleased with this display of love and cheer.

As we gathered around in a circle, my niece Kim's husband, Allen Pete, gave the invocation before we proceeded to eat. At this time, I announced to the 30+ in attendance, my news of writing this book. I asked Elroy to tell them the title of the book and he told them that the name of the book was "The Ultimate Surprise" and everybody applauded and gave lots of hugs of congratulations. They were amazed that I had accomplished this feat, as well as all of my friends, after having a brain tumor and surgery. To sit down and write a book was next to amazing to everybody and they were mainly in shock that their sister, aunt and grandmother could do this. I sometimes shock myself when I am writing yet another chapter. I don't think I am amazing, but I think of myself as being blessed and having a lot of faith in God.

To have family that love and care for you is special and I am blessed to have that foundation. Even though while growing up, we were all we had. There were no family reunions for us because we were our only family members. We were small then, but our family is growing with each new birth or marriage. That makes us strong and able to conquer any obstacle that is in our way. We are well connected and hope that we stay that way.

CHAPTER 21

Holidays
(Thanksgiving, Christmas, New Year)

With our Thanksgiving Day, we were very thankful for my presence and being able to prepare Thanksgiving dinner. My daughter, Jameka and granddaughter, Adrianna, came from North Carolina to share dinner with us. They didn't stay all day because Jameka had to get back so she could go shopping on Black Friday. I didn't mind, though, as long as she came to visit us on this special day. We were all thankful for me being here and still doing better. The pain is still present as well as the numbness in my face, but it is bearable. When you have so much pain constantly, you learn to deal with it as if it is just a part of your life. I look at my pain like that and sometimes when I hurt, I try to conceal it and keep it to myself with the exception when Elroy has his watchful eye on my facial expression and figure out that I am hurting. I can't hide anything from him even though at this time, it is 7 months since the surgery. It makes me wonder if the pain will ever go away. Deep down inside, I know that it will and I must be patient. I've learned that patience is a virtue and I'm dealing with that each and every day as I feel the pain.

Christmas was extra special for us. We were not able to exchange gifts but Elroy told me that I was his present because I was there with him and he was very thankful for that. He did not want any other gifts. He said his Christmas came in April and that was enough for him. We just praised the Lord and thanked Him, again, for blessing us and for me being here to enjoy the birth of Jesus Christ. December 25 marked the 8th month since my surgery. I had my surgery on April 25. This was a very blessed event for us and we got through this holiday just fine. Jameka and Adrianna came to visit on Christmas Eve and that was very exciting because to see family on special holidays means a lot to me because I am a very family oriented person and I just love my family. Any chance to see a family member is very special. So, we were thankful to have friends who cared for us and assisted us with Christmas dinner and other necessities we needed for the holiday. They will always be remembered and appreciated for their kindness. We are fortunate to have such dear friends. To be able to celebrate this holiday and not in as much pain was a reminder of the "ultimate surprise" and how it was fading from our memory and conversations. We know that it will always be in our thoughts but not as vivid as it was 8 months ago. We'll never forget this surprise but we won't keep dwelling on it either. If it decides to just go away into oblivion, we won't mind one bit. As a matter of fact, we will wish it a bon voyage on its journey into oblivion.

The New Year holiday was another blessed event. I had to work New Year's Eve but Elroy had that day off. As a matter of fact, it was not as bad as I thought going to work on that day, because it was very quiet, but also busy. I really did not mind being there since I knew I would be off the next day, which was New Year's Day and I could get some rest. The New Year came in very quiet for us but we were able to toast it together and prayed that God, again, allowed me to be here to see this New Year and we were very grateful. We saw the ball drop in Times Square and were very excited to see that once again.

We realized that this ultimate surprise was with us for the new year and we prayed that it won't see another year. That was our wish that we hope will be granted and come true for us. NO MORE "ULTIMATE SURPRISE", EVER!!

CHAPTER 22

Things I Miss

While recovering from this ultimate surprise, there were things that I missed doing, especially during the summer months. I will list them:

- Cooking on the grill

- Being able to care for outdoor plants

- Shopping

- Getting hair & nails done

- Going out to dinner

- Preparing meals

- Housework (well, I really don't miss this, but what can I say?)

- Driving (The waiting game is getting unbearable at times)

- I miss being who I was before the surgery

I feel that once I am back to myself, these things that I miss will come back into play and I will be able to do anything I want to do without limitations. Well, there may be some limitations since I will still have the affects of this ultimate surprise. These affects will be with me at least for another year, especially the healing of the skull. It is still very tender around the incision area and it hurts really bad sometimes, but it will also get better when the time is right. This is something that you can't rush because all the healing process is on a time table and that time table cannot be disturbed or disrupted. That is the way it is and it will definitely take more time to heal. I can be patient just knowing how the outcome will be after this is all said and done. I have faith in my surgeon, myself and modern medicine.

CHAPTER 23

Almost One Year Later

As I approach the one-year mark of this "ultimate surprise", I can honestly say that things are much improved. The light is shining at the end of the tunnel. It's still a little dull, but I am hopeful that as each day progresses, it will shine brighter. There are still episodes of nerve discomfort but I am unable to take medication for it because of the side effects I suffered while taking three different nerve medicines to find the right one. I am convinced that there is no right one for me. It wasn't good, but you have to look at the big picture, though. The medicine was used to treat one symptom and in the meantime, it gave me some totally new symptons that had to be treated. Go figure! Modern medicine! In my case, though, I take so many different medications that I wonder how the doctors can tell which medicines are giving me the side effects. I read all the pamphlets that come with each medication and I can pretty well pin point which medicines are causing me the discomforts. Those pamphlets are very good reading material as long as you don't try to make something out of nothing. It is some very helpful information and much needed to keep you informed about what you are putting in your body.

My visit with the Oncologist in March went very well and he was amazed at how good I look. It seems that I get this from everybody I come in contact with who knows about the surgery. It makes me wonder how I looked before the surgery. It is a good feeling to know that I don't look sickly and frail but the picture of good health. Well, maybe not good health but healthy looking. The doctor advised me that I will have to get MRIs for the rest of my life to make sure there are no more "ultimate surprises" hiding in my head. I would hate to go through this ordeal again, so rest assured that I will get those MRIs done when advised to do so. He scheduled another appointment to see me in six months. That will be interesting. The radiation treatments slowed down the progression of the tail that was left from the tumor but we don't know how much since the last MRI was taken in December. I go back to see the surgeon in June and hopefully, he will order one before the appointment. This ultimate surprise should rest in peace and become a figment of my imagination for the rest of my life.

I started back driving on March 16, 2009 and the experience wasn't as bad as I thought. I was very nervous for the first week, but now I am able to go with the flow of the traffic and reach my destination without any problem. It is truly a blessing to get that part of my independence back and not have to rely on people to take me places. I still like for Elroy to transport me around on the weekends and he loves doing it. It seems that he is having a problem letting go and want to keep me helpless, but I am showing him every day that I am really getting better and can do some things for myself. He'll soon realize this and give me a little more space to grow back into myself before this ultimate surprise invaded our space. That day is coming.

On April 20, 2009, I will officially start working 8 hours a day. I have been working 7 hours a day so one more hour shouldn't make that much difference. This will surely be a challenge for the first few weeks because my system is used to shutting down around 5:30 p.m. in the evening. It's amazing how your body gets used to being one way and takes its time accepting change. Getting off at 4:00 p.m. allowed me to get the rest I needed during that period of time, but since I will be getting off at 5:00 p.m., I have to retrain my body to stay awake a little longer. This is something else that I know I can do. At this point in my life, I feel that I can do almost anything. To be able to get back in a routine was something I didn't think would happen one year ago but I can honestly say, "look at me now". The feel of being me is slowly returning and I like that feeling.

This ultimate surprise was not expected or wanted but it was there and with all the prayers sent out for me, it will just be a reminder of what it was and no more. Life throws different curves at you to make you aware of what's in store for you and how to cope with different obstacles. To have faith in God and what He can do for you will help you conquer those obstacles and see your life in a different light. It truly made a believer out of me. The power of prayer is awesome.

I am so fortunate to be given a second chance in life and I am looking forward to spending more time with my friends and family. To enjoy my grandchildren and watch them grow into adulthood is what I'm really looking forward to because they are a part of me and I love them very much. It's a blessing to have children and grandchildren because you can see yourself in them and want them to have a better life than you had. I am happy that my daughters have a better life than I had and that makes me very proud of the young ladies they have become as mothers. They are good mothers but I am the best mother to them and they know that for a fact.

CHAPTER 24

Epilogue

I would like to thank you for reading this book. I felt that this was something that I had to do to make everyone know that because you are diagnosed with a brain tumor, it is not necessarily the end of your life, the end of the world or a death wish. With today's most modern medical technology and skilled surgeons, there is proof that tumors can be surgically removed and they are not always cancerous. It depends on where the tumor is located and the type of tumor that it is. Meningiomas are very rarely cancerous and I was very fortunate that was the type that I had. Now, having a tumor is not being fortunate, but a non-cancerous one is very fortunate for the individual. Still, it is not anything to make light of because it is an invasion in your body. The body can reject this invasion and that is when the symptons flare up. The only thing about a brain tumor removal is the painful recovery. It is pain that you just can't describe because it is so severe, intense and excruciating, but with lots of prayer, proper medication, a loving and caring husband, as well as family and friends, and a very caring surgeon, that makes everything, including the pain, easier to bear.

If you should have an unusual headache, seek medical attention. All headaches are not migraines. Listen to that little voice and hope that you won't have an ultimate surprise, but if you do have that surprise, take it very seriously and listen to your doctors. They are trained to help you and make sure that your ultimate surprise won't hang around long. It will be eradicated and become a thing of the past. Please listen to me and do what the doctor tell you to do because they will make you much better. I am living proof of that as I write this book for you.

As I close this chapter, I am looking forward to the day when the nerves in my face finally realize they are alive and wake up. I am looking forward to the day when Dr. Koen will tell me that there is no more tumor; it is gone. What a wonderful day that will be. I am looking forward to the day that I am back to myself one hundred percent again and able to do daily activities, besides going to work. I want to be able to do normal things around the house and to go shopping by myself. I want to do these things myself and I am sure that day will soon be here when totally dependency will be just for me.

The year 2008 will be a memory but I will never forget "The Ultimate Surprise". It is now 2009, so I know things are going to be better. I have lots to look forward to and when those days finally come to pass, I will rejoice and "The Ultimate Surprise" will be no more.

The impact I felt and faced from this ultimate surprise:

- Stress

- Trying to Survive

- Job Situation

- Finances

- The Traumatic Situation

- Unexpected

- Pain that continues after 8 months

- Radiation Treatments

- Nerve Damage

- More medication for the nerves in my face

- Trials and Tribulations each and every day, but still have the faith to get through these obstacles.

- Incapacitated but with God's blessing, Elroy was able to strive and took everyday in stride because he knew he had the Lord on his side and without Him he could not have made it.

Elroy's final words:

"Thank the Lord for everything. He's a good God. I thank Him that you are still here with me through the trials and tribulations. It's a blessing to be in good health to take care of you". "I am proud of you, my little Grasshopper". These are his words that he wanted included in this "Ultimate Surprise."

Keep praying for me.

Thank you.

ACKNOWLEDGMENTS

I would like to dedicate this book to, first, God Almighty, which I never would have made it without Him. My husband, Elroy Jones, provided the best care than any doctor or health care personnel could have given to me during this ordeal from beginning to the present. He is a constant reminder of true love and dedication to your significant other. My daughters, Jameka Patrick and Jacqueline Wilson provided me with extra strength to get better. My 3 grandchildren, Adrianna Smith, Xavier and Joshua Wilson for their unwavering love for their "Grammy" and my son-in-law, Adam Wilson, for being instrumental in helping my daughter and grandsons make the trip from Washington State to Virginia to be by my side before, during and after surgery.

I have several friends and guardian angels to thank, also. For several months, Jim Keithan, the IT Technician at work, provided me transportation to work without being asked. He definitely was heaven sent. In this day and time, people like him are very rare. By the way, I work for the Norfolk Airport Authority® as an Executive Administrative Assistant to the Executive Director, Kenneth R. Scott and Deputy Executive Director, Wayne E. Shank. I must say that they are the best employers this side of heaven. They continue to work with me and my reduced hours at work and they never complain. I am very thankful to have them as my bosses because they are very compassionate and understanding. I've never heard them utter a negative word since I've been going through this ordeal. It makes you wonder why you are in the presence of such wonderful employers. I don't have to wonder any further because I know why I am in their presence.

Other co-workers who showed love and support were Debra Moss, Diane Edwards (who serves as my mother hen), Rose Marie Iervolino who made sure I get to my office safely in the mornings,

Lynne Westermeyer who works for US Airways and Mr. William Jones, the Finance Director, who also assisted in rides to work. Michelle Rogers, who is our "Plant Lady" provided transportation to me as well and still offers me words of encouragement. Diane's daughter, Gale Edwards, provided assistance in taking me to my early radiation treatments, waiting for me afterwards and taking me back to work. She also tried to assist me in getting transportation to the remainder of my treatments. I had a network of friends to offer assistance to me and for that I am forever grateful and thankful.

My transportation to my radiation treatments was fulfilled by these ladies who I have to collectively thank: Laura Barnes, Susan Bates, Jeanne Earley, Diane Dempsey, Debra Sessoms, Debbie Meads, Bonnie Sampere, Janet Rial and Betty Ann Gravely. Even though all of these ladies did not physically provide the actual transportation, they were available as back-ups in case the other ladies had unforeseen circumstances. It is better to be prepared for the unknown and the unexpected. It was just amazing to see the love that was being generated from my friends. They are really true friends and I love and thank them very much and they will always have a special place in my heart. They really lived up to the saying, "if you need anything, just call." It was a call that I did not want to make, but need makes you do those things that you would not normally do and that is what I did. To see them come to my rescue so quickly was truly remarkable and very much appreciated.

I cannot forget my neighbor, Amanda Stoewer, who is in the Navy. She gave me rides home while she was working at Naval Station Norfolk and I was working 4 hours a day. She was getting off at noon and was able to pick me up with no problem because the airport was not out of her way. My other neighbors, the Wilsons, were very neighborly in showing their concern for me and my husband. Their concern for my husband as well as for me was far and beyond what neighbors do for neighbors and their care and concern will never be forgotten.

For all of my friends who sent cards and flowers while I was recuperating, I want to thank you, too. It is too numerous to name everybody for their kindness but I wanted to still acknowledge your thoughtfulness and to let you know how much it was very much appreciated. All thoughts and prayers during this time were needed and received. All acts of kindness will never be forgotten.

A special thank you to Dr. Joseph Koen and his surgical team for removing this "ultimate surprise" and taking very good care of me. To have a surgeon with a caring attitude, perfect bedside manners and his only concern is for your well being is astronomical. I was very fortunate that my primary care physician referred me to him. He already knew that I would get the very best care possible. Dr. Koen has a gentle way about him that emits to his patients. I could see that in him during my very first visit. He listens very carefully to my concerns and answers my question very frankly. He does not sugar coat anything that he says to me and, I guess, that could be a good thing sometimes. We, as humans, sometimes can't handle the truth but have to when it affects our lives. He has a way to saying things that make you think and understand what he is saying to you. I was glad that my daughter and husband were in his presence when he spoke these things because they understood what he was saying better than I did at the time. As time went on and the ultimate surprise was removed, I could understand more of what he was saying and appreciated what he was saying. What a difference the removal of this ultimate surprise made in our lives.

I was not happy with the "ultimate surprise" but was pleased with its removal even though the healing process was very painful. Almost one year later, I can still feel the effects of it through the nerve discomfort and the pain at the incision while the skull heals. I am very happy, though, that Dr. Koen was there every step of the way and continues to be a part of my life.

Thank you, again, Dr. Koen

The passageway through life is filled with turmoil, but while walking through this passageway, you pick up friends along the way to guide you. The Ultimate Surprise might be that passageway for a stranger who is seeking resistance from such turmoil. Please pay attention to the little signs that are guiding you and do not take any detours. These signs were placed in your path for a reason. Don't look the other way, but please read and follow the signs.

Once again, I want to thank everyone that played a part in this "Ultimate Surprise".

www.ingramcontent.com/pod-product-compliance
Lightning Source LLC
Chambersburg PA
CBHW031304280526
45784CB00004B/1979